MUSTARD PLASTERS AND HANDCARS

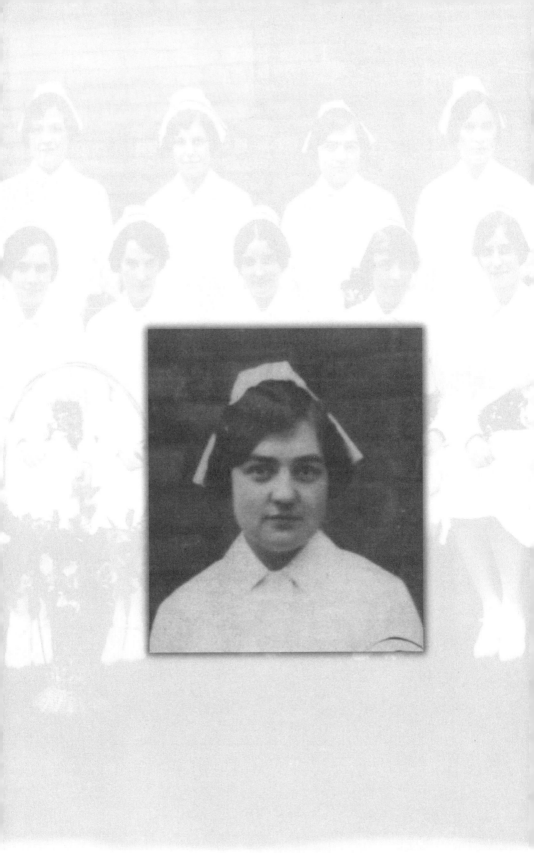

MUSTARD PLASTERS AND HANDCARS

THROUGH THE EYES OF A RED CROSS OUTPOST NURSE

GERTRUDE LeROY MILLER

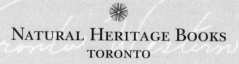

NATURAL HERITAGE BOOKS
TORONTO

*...For the dedicated women who served so well as Red Cross
Outpost Nurses in isolated rural communities of Canada.*

Published by Natural Heritage/Natural History Inc.
P.O. Box 95, Station O, Toronto, Ontario M4A 2M8

Design by Blanche Hamill, Norton Hamill Design
Edited by Jane Gibson
Printed and bound in Canada by Hignell Printing Limited

Canadian Cataloguing in Publication Data

Miller, Gertrude LeRoy, 1902–1983
Mustard plasters and handcars: through the eyes of a red cross outpost nurse

Includes bibliographical references and index.
ISBN 1-896219-65-9

1. Miller, Gertrude LeRoy, 1902–1983. 2. Red Cross Outpost Hospital
(Wilberforce,Ont.)–History 3. Wilberforce (Ont. : Township)–Social conditions.
4. Public health nurses–Ontario–Wilberforce (Township)–Biography. I. Title

RT37.M54A3 2000   610.73'4'092   C00-931211-0

THE CANADA COUNCIL | LE CONSEIL DES ARTS
FOR THE ARTS | DU CANADA
SINCE 1957 | DEPUIS 1957

Natural Heritage/Natural History Inc. acknowledges the support received for its publishing program from the Canada Council Block Grant Program and the assistance of
the Association for the Export of Canadian Books, Ottawa. Natural Heritage also
acknowledges the support of the Ontario Council for the Arts for its publishing program.

Preface

The story goes that just before 3:00 a.m. on March 13, 1933, my mother rang the bedside bell and called upstairs to the nurse. Minutes later at 3:03 a.m. I made my first appearance at the Wilberforce Red Cross Outpost Hospital.

Gertrude LeRoy, the resident Red Cross Nurse awoke in her room upstairs. Quickly, she lit the kerosene lamp, alerted her only assistant, the young housekeeper, Aileen Ames, readied herself and hurried downstairs to take care of her patient.

Yes, the nurse lived at the hospital. The Outpost was her home as well as her workplace. Twenty-four hours a day, seven days a week, with only a few weeks of holiday each year, she was always on call. Sometimes patients came to her. Sometimes she went to them in their homes. She visited the schools to check the health of the children and taught the importance of hygiene and prevention of disease. The Red Cross Outpost Nurse was an integral part of the community, a participant in the daily life of the village.

Red Cross Outpost Nurses? Outpost Hospitals? What was this Red Cross Outpost Hospital service? How did it begin?

In the early 1920s, leaders of the Canadian Red Cross in Toronto were recognizing that in many isolated rural communities in Canada there was little or no medical service available. Many people were miles away from the over-worked country doctors. Hospitals were mainly far away in citites. The Red Cross had proven its organizational and medical abilities in the recently ended Great War of 1914-1918. Perhaps it could step into the breach in peacetime and somehow help provide health services in rural areas.

At this very time Alfred Schofield of Wilberforce, Ontario, contacted them, requesting some medical help for the folks in his home area. The Red Cross was responsive and ready. Their requirements were straight-forward. Provide a building for a hospital in your village. Furnish the

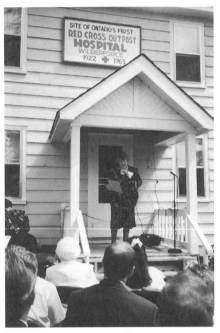

Hilda Clark speaking at the opening of the Wilberforce Red Cross Outpost Museum.

building, heat it and make it live-able. The Red Cross would employ a nurse, acquire some supplies and begin providing health services.

Armed with this information, Mr. Schofield returned to Wilberforce in Monmouth Township, Haliburton County, where he was the Children's Aid Society Officer. Perceiving this response to be an excellent opportunity, five leading citizens of Monmouth formed a corporation and, on behalf of the people of the surrounding area, they acquired a two-story house in Wilberforce. Thanks to them, to the Canadian Red Cross and to the many other hard-working volunteers, this building became the *first* Red Cross Outpost Hospital in Ontario. In February 1922 with the arrival of nurse, Miss Josephine Jackson, the Outpost Hospital Service began in earnest.

By the time Gertrude LeRoy arrived in September 1930, six nurses had, in turn, served the health needs of the people of Wilberforce and area. By then, over twenty-five Red Cross Outpost Hospitals had been established in rural Ontario communities and more would be added. How welcome this health/medical service proved to be to many grateful people.

Records indicate that close to sixty babies were born in Monmouth Township between February 1922 and 1930 with the Outpost nurse in attendance. Sometimes a doctor would be present, but frequently the nurse was on her own. Some babies were born at home, some at the Outpost. Like all of her predecessors, Miss LeRoy had gained much experience in maternity cases after her arrival in Wilberforce in September 1930. By the time of my birth two and half years later, she was a much practised pro.

This book, Gertrude's story of her four years as nurse in charge of

Preface

our Outpost, includes many accounts of how she helped deliver a range of health services, particulary the aid in maternity cases. Her tales of travelling to the homes of patients, often being conveyed on the railway handcar and other now outdated modes of transportation, coping with winter snows and spring mud, are spun throughout the book.

This publication of the author's recollections of her experiences as a Red Cross Outpost Nurse and her impressions of the challenges, the difficulties and joys of rural life in our part of Ontario, Canada, is a much appreciated record of one aspect of our history. It is hoped that people in this area, nurses of all ages and fields of interest, and the family and friends of the late Gertrude LeRoy Miller, as well as people with a general interest in Ontario history will treasure and celebrate this book. Gertrude was there at my birth. I value and celebrate having some part in the safe delivery, in book form, of her story, *Mustard Plasters and Handcars: Through the Eyes of a Red Cross Outpost Nurse.*

Hilda G. J. Clark
Past President, Wilberforce Heritage Guild

Contents

Introduction

Mustard Plasters and Handcars: Through the Eyes of a Red Cross Outpost Nurse presents details, impressions, and glimpses of life in earlier times in our area. Central to this story by Gertrude LeRoy Miller is Ontario's *first* Red Cross Outpost Hospital in Wilberforce where the author served as nurse-in-charge from September 1930 to the end of August 1934. The Outpost is also central to the Wilberforce Heritage Guild which was formed in March 1991 to preserve that historic building and other aspects of local history.

Until the establishment of the Wilberforce Outpost in 1922, the scattered population of a few hundred in this area depended on each other's practical knowledge and skills for medical/health care assistance, and the few doctors (G.P.s) who had ventured here of their own accord or with the encouragement of lumbering or mining companies.

By the time the author arrived as an enthusiastic, recently graduated public health nurse, Monmouth Township, in Haliburton County, where Wilberforce is located, had been incorporated (1881) as a municipality for fifty years. Settlers had straggled into the area to take up land grants beginning in 1871 when the township was first surveyed and with the building of the Burleigh and Monck colonization roads. They carved out a living mainly by farming on the rocky, hilly terrain, and working for lumber companies who had rights to the most valuable timber in the area.

When the much needed Red Cross Outpost Hospital and nursing service began, the Irondale, Bancroft and Ottawa Railway (I.B.&O.) had been in operation through the area for about twenty-five years. With the railway, came the railway telephone which was often used to contact doctors in Bancroft, Haliburton village and beyond.

At the convenient intersection of the I.B.&O. rail line and the Burleigh Road, people had gradually set up businesses and homes, then a school, a church and a hall. A post office opened, listed as

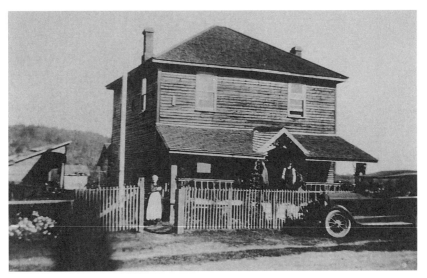

The Wilberforce Red Cross Outpost Hospital being prepared for use in the early 1920s. The building, originally owned by John Holmes, was purchased by Alfred Fleming. He sold the building to Monmouth Charitable Association in 1924 for $650. The building was in public use since it opened as an Outpost Hospital until 1963. Today it is a museum once more open to the public. *Courtesy Wilberforce Heritage Guild.*

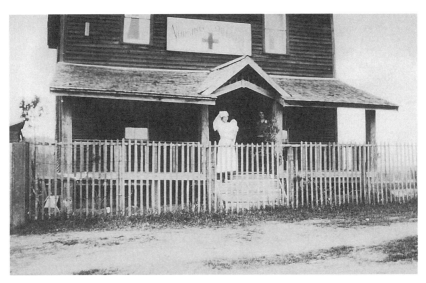

Miss Catherine Lawrence holding the first baby born at the Outpost May 1924. Mrs. George Barnes who was President at the time is the other lady in the picure, and the baby (Hugh) is the son of Mr. & Mrs. Fred Perry. *Courtesy Wilberforce Heritage Guild.*

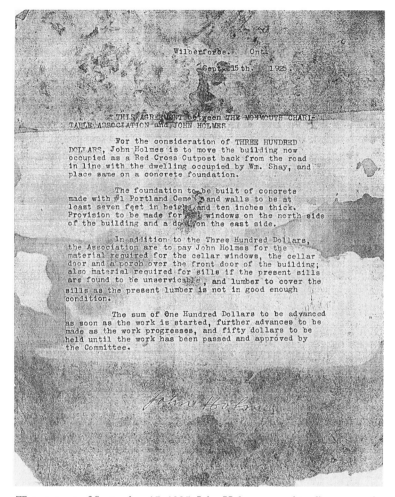

The contract of September 15, 1925. John Holmes agreed to dig a new cellar, build a foundation and move the whole Outpost building back from the edge of the road, closer to the lake, as well as make other improvements. *Courtesy Wilberforce Heritage Guild.*

Pusey, named after Charles Pusey, an I.B.&O. official. Since many of the residents had gravitated to this location from the original Wilberforce settlement which had centred around Poverty (later Wilbermere) Lake, a few kilometres to the south, the name Wilberforce moved with them and soon officially replaced the name Pusey. Wilberforce proudly takes its name from William Wilberforce, the legislator who introduced the Anti-Slave Trade legislation into the British Parliament.

Many of Gertrude LeRoy's nursing adventures related in this book describe her activities with patients and others outside Wilberforce since the Red Cross Outpost nurses served the people of Essonville, Hadlington, Hotspur and Tory Hill, other communities that had developed in Monmouth Township. Residents of Highland Grove and Cheddar in nearby Cardiff Township, Harcourt and Kennaway in Dysart et al., and Gooderham in Glamorgan Township benefitted from and supported this service as well.

Throughout the book, Gertrude LeRoy Miller portrays how isolated this area was, even 60 years after the arrival of the first settlers. She describes just how scattered the small population was, and yet how self-sufficient many residents tended to be, always willing to help others, identifying needs and raising funds for important causes such as the Outpost Hospital. This publication not only furthers the Wilberforce Heritage Guild's goal of preserving stories of our past, but it is our hope that it will stimulate interest in the Outpost in its present role as a museum. The presence of this historic house is a place of pride for residents, and one of interest to those visiting our area as tourists. As well, the book adds to the historical record of the Red Cross in its development and operation of the Outpost Hospital service from 1922 until the 1970s, and of its valuable benefit to Canadians. Just as in Halburton County, many rural communities had no hospitals until the Red Cross established their Oupost hospitals in their areas.

The publication of *Mustard Plasters and Handcars: Through the Eyes of a Red Cross Outpost Nurse* celebrates Gertrude LeRoy Miller's work as a Red Cross Outpost Nurse, her leadership abilities, her considerable creative artistic talents and her determination to write this story of an important part of her life. It celebrates, as well, the achievements and contributions of all the young Red Cross Outpost Nurses who provided much needed health and medical help in many isolated rural Canadian communities, while also acknowledging the exceptional demands made on them as professionals.

We are indebted to the author for her detailed, delightful and forthright account of four years, and more, of the history of Wilberforce and surrounding area. Current and former directors of the Wilberforce Heritage Guild, whose efforts have resulted in the publication of this book sincerely believe that Gertrude LeRoy Miller's story, her sketches, and her paintings are clearly artistic and cultural expressions of the history of our community, our way of life, our heritage. May this book inspire its readers to know and appreciate their past, and to realize that they too can welcome and meet challenges and opportunities in the future. Would that the author were alive to celebrate with us, the publication of her *Mustard Plasters and Handcars: Through the Eyes of a Red Cross Outpost Nurse.*

Directors, Past and Present
Wilberforce Heritage Guild

Cathy Agnew, Hilda Clark, Lloyd Griffiths, Margaret Harrison, Ernie Hemphill, Judy Johnson, Marlene Robertson, Kenneth Sanderson, Nadeen Sanderson, Gerald Shackleton, Patricia Simiana, Gloria Solmes, Gillian Stephen, Florence Taylor, June Williams. From Original Board: Winnie Schofield, Publicity, and the late Harry Clark representing Monmouth Township Council.

MUSTARD PLASTERS
AND HANDCARS

1

Not a Stranger for Long

Time: 5:00 a.m., Sunday, September 14, 1930

A Model T, motor running and with a strange man at the wheel, waited at the gate in the haze of early dawn. Up in my room, by the yellow light of a kerosene lamp, I rummaged through my trunk in search of clothing suitable for a mysterious trip into the unknown.

Normally, a young woman would hesitate before accepting such an invitation, especially at 5 a.m., but not I! I was thrilled! This was my first exciting step toward the great adventure for which I had been preparing these past four years and, I hoped, a taste of what lay ahead. Four days ago I had arrived at this one nurse Red Cross Outpost as a Registered Nurse. With my brand new diploma in Public Health Nursing in my trunk, along with books and notebooks full of health rules and directions for their application, I was bursting with energy and desire to use them.

Four years and three months earlier I had dedicated my life to the service of my fellow human beings, under the direction of the Great Physician. From that time on, many incidents happened which convinced me that I was being divinely guided toward a nursing career. Even the awarding of a scholarship to study Public Health Nursing at the University of Toronto seemed to be a sign. During my time there, I had a chance to visit the Red Cross Headquarters where I met Maude Wilkinson, Assistant Director and Ruby Hamilton, Nursing

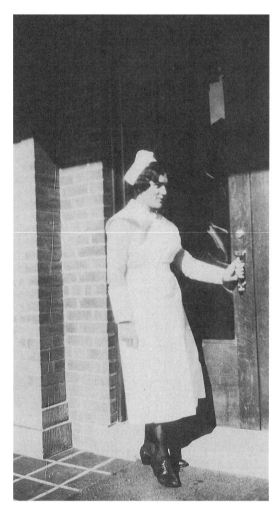

In 1929, Gertrude LeRoy graduated as a Registered Nurse at Toronto Western Hospital. Here she is shown outside the Nurse's Residence. *Courtesy Virginia (LeRoy) Luckock, sister of Gertrude.*

Supervisor. That visit resulted in my being asked to come to Wilberforce, where I would be in "complete charge" of the Red Cross Outpost, the first to be opened in Ontario.

My assigned location was situated in the quiet little village of Wilberforce, which had a population of about 200. With that as my headquarters, I would work throughout the area, attending the sick in their homes as well as those who came to the Outpost for treatment or care. There, too, I would give first aid in emergencies. There would be considerable amount of maternity work, but doctors were within calling distance. Also, there were twelve schools to be visited twice a year, if possible, to carry out a general Public Health Program. The

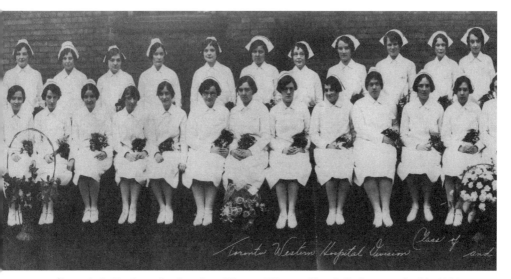

Gertrude LeRoy's graduating class (Toronto Western Hospital) photographed in 1929. Gertrude is the third nurse from the left in the back row. *Courtesy Donna Miller Fry, granddaughter of Gertrude LeRoy Miller.*

Outpost would be my home and I would have a housekeeper who would look after my needs. I should have some spare time to relax and enjoy a hobby or two, it was said. Miss Wilkinson warned me that winters "up there" were extremely cold and that a fur coat was practically a "must." A fur coat! That was something I hadn't even dreamed of. She hastened to assure me, however, that it would not be necessary for me to purchase a car until spring (something else I hadn't counted on). It would be impossible to use a car during the winter and spring months because of snow and mud conditions. In the meantime, I would hire transportation.

Wednesday, September 10 arrived very suddenly, it seemed. My trunk was packed and I was on my way. While purchasing my ticket at Union Station [in Toronto] about 9 a.m., I was asked by the agent if I had ever been to Wilberforce before. When I told him I hadn't even heard of the place until recently, he said he had been up that way fishing and that it was beautiful country. He then told me I would have plenty of time to admire the scenery on my way.

It wasn't until late afternoon, that the significance of that remark became clear. According to the schedule, we were to arrive in Wilberforce at 4:30 p.m., but at that time we were nowhere near the place. I was very thankful to have heeded Miss Hamilton's advice and packed a good substantial lunch.

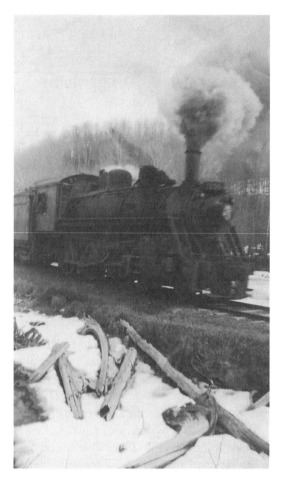

The Irondale, Bancroft and Ottawa (I.B.&.O.) Railway engine producing great smoke as it chugged into Wilberforce, circa early 1940s. Construction of this line began eastward from Howland Junction in 1883 and from mile 20.1, halfway between Gooderham and Tory Hill, in December 1894. It would likely have extended to Wilberforce within the next two years. The first I.B.&O. train to reach Bancroft arrived there on September 12, 1910. *Courtesy Hilda Clark Collection.*

I had changed trains in Lindsay and was now riding an old-fashioned plush-seated coach with no more than a dozen other passengers, the only passenger car at the end of a long string of boxcars. Evidently this railway line depended more on freight than passengers. The pot-bellied stove at one end of the coach was, of course, not in use this beautiful September day, but at the rate we were travelling it might well be needed before the end of the journey. Many changes could take place during this trip into the northern wilderness.

Although well supplied with reading material, I found it more fascinating to gaze out of the window and watch the ever-changing landscape of hills and streams, evergreens and beautiful white birch. Occasionally there were brief stops at small stations where mailbags were

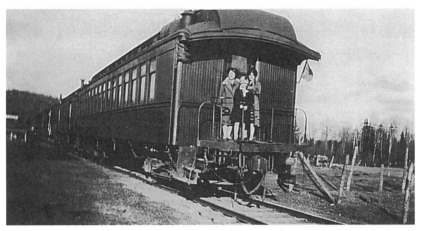

An I.B.&O. railway coach about 1926. *Photo by Marjorie (Cronsberry) Pollock, donated to the Wilberforce Heritage Guild Collection by Aileen (Young) Broughton.*

exchanged and often some freight. The sameness of the hours was altered, however, when suddenly we stopped, seemingly in the middle of nowhere. I could hear the engine shunting. One of the passengers informed me that this was Howland Junction, where the line branched, one leg going northwest to Haliburton and the other northeast to Bancroft. Wilberforce was on the Bancroft line. Here at the junction we would change engines, the one coming from Bancroft would turn around, pick up our train and go back, while our engine would turn around and take the cars from Bancroft to Lindsay. We all watched as each engine in turn was driven slowly onto a round platform, called a turntable. Once in place, the train crews put their weight to the bars around the edge and pushed it around, positioning the locomotives for their new runs. Soon we were on our way once more.

From that point on the scenery seemed more beautiful than ever. The hills were so much higher, the rocks and streams more numerous. I was fascinated by the sight of the engine away ahead on the curves, chugging its way in and out among the hills and around ponds like the head of a giant serpent. Behind the head trailed its body of red box cars. Then the head would disappear from view as a steep hill or rock cut or thick woods loomed up, hiding it momentarily. A jolt, a sway, a few harsh screeches and my view would be obstructed by a wall of solid rock or tall evergreens. I was thankful for our slow pace for not only was I enjoying the scenery, but any greater speed would surely derail us on one of those sharp curves.

Actually, this was much like the very type of country I had often dreamed of exploring. Now that dream was coming true. One thing I decided; there was no shortage of subjects to paint[1] during some of that spare time I'd been promised. However, the purpose of this trip was to serve humanity. What if this was only 150 miles from home? It would be just temporary. Didn't Miss Hamilton say it was an emergency? No doubt in a few months I would be sent farther afield,[2] where I could apply my nursing skills.

At last, when my watch told me it was 6:30, two hours later than scheduled, the conductor swung down the aisle calling, "Next stop, Wilberforce!" Only three other passengers remained besides myself. As the train drew up to the station, I seemed to be the only one making a move to get off, but the large crowd of people on the station platform caught my curiosity. I decided that a very important person must have been waiting to come aboard.

As I stepped off the coach, a very pleasant looking young woman, introducing herself as the nurse[3] whom I had come to replace, greeted me. I was so excited I paid no attention to the crowd, which the nurse also ignored as she led me quickly to her car. "Don't bother about your luggage," she said, "It will be looked after."

As we drove away, I ventured to ask her the reason for the large crowd. "They've come to get a glimpse of the new nurse," she said. "You'll notice as we drive through town, those who didn't come to the station will either be in their front yards or peeking from behind their curtains." They were. Well, didn't my chest expand! For once in my life I was a V.I.P.! Imagine everyone in town turning out to see me!

As it was only a short drive to the Outpost, I did not have much of an opportunity to get the lay of land. I noticed a row of houses on our left, all surrounded by wire fences. A general store, a mill yard and a couple of houses were on the right. One, a large stone house, had a Post Office sign over the front door. Then we stopped in front of the most decrepit looking building of them all. It had evidently been painted white at one time, but not the ugly box-like structure[4] stuck on the front, which had been put up, I suppose, to keep out the snow in the winter. However, a large white freshly-painted sign hanging overhead left no doubt in a weary traveller's mind about this being the "Red Cross Outpost."

It is difficult to remember just exactly what my feelings were when we stopped at this sad-looking building. I think they were somewhere between disappointment and pity. So this was supposed to be a small

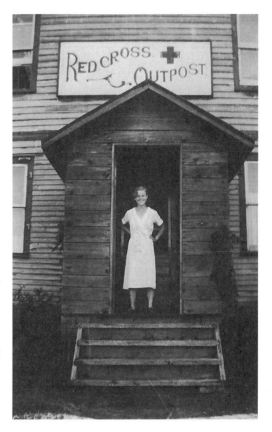

Aileen Ames, though only in her early teens, had already been the housekeeper at the Wilberforce Outpost for a year when Gertrude LeRoy arrived. She worked there from 1929 to 1936. Aileen's recent comment about this picture: "I look as if I owned the place!" Apparently Aileen made the Outpost a very "happy" place for both the nurse and the patients. *Donated to Wilberforce Heritage Guild Collection by Aileen Ames Walker.*

hospital! My idea of a hospital, small or large, was of a neat freshly painted and attractive building. This community must indeed need help!

The nurse opened the squeaky gate and we walked up the gravel path to the steep rough plank steps. A sweet looking young girl was waiting at the door and the nurse introduced her as Aileen,[5] the housekeeper. Housekeeper! What could a young girl like that know about housekeeping, especially in a hospital? I was soon to find out.

Once through the door we passed into a narrow hall; a closed stairway was on the right. On a high shelf on the left wall squatted a stubby coal oil lamp with a reflector behind it. Evidently our bright light! That was another matter that hadn't entered my mind. How could I ever get used to this kind of illumination after the bright lights of the city hospital?

The hall led to a large room stretching the full width of the building. At either end was a narrow window covered with "lace" curtains that had seen better days. The lower three or so feet of the walls were trimmed with wood wainscotting painted dark brown. The upper walls and ceiling were covered with buff paper, which here and there had cracked and curled up, exposing rough boards.[6] A black stovepipe protruded through the floor near the kitchen door, which was directly opposite the hall, and continued on up through the ceiling. The floor was covered with badly worn and cracked linoleum also painted brown.

One end of this room served as living room and office and contained furniture looking like discards: an oversize flat top desk, a steel cot covered with faded chintz, a couple of wicker chairs and a set of shelves which must have been built by an amateur carpenter using odds and ends of boards of various lengths and thickness. These were set into a corner and were filled with books, also discards.

The other end of the room served as a dining area with a round table and a set of four chairs, the best-looking furniture so far. The table was covered with a snow-white cloth and neatly set with odd dishes.

A delicious hot meal was waiting for the three of us. Although I had been nibbling on sandwiches and fruit for the last eight or nine hours, I really did enjoy the dinner. It was especially thoughtful for them to have waited to eat with me.

While we were still at the table, two husky young men arrived with my trunk and other luggage. After being introduced as Lorne and Earle,[7] they carried the things upstairs and left. A tour of the building came next. Before it was completed, I had decided that Aileen had been wise to serve such an enjoyable dinner first.

The kitchen was bright and new. This, I was told, had been built onto the back of the main building two years ago, replacing an old shed. It was the pride and joy of the community, with its modern cupboards with sliding doors (which I found seldom slid). There were several large deep drawers which never worked properly either. The kitchen even boasted a white enamelled sink, at the end of which stood the source of water supply, the pump. I was soon to learn that a great amount of human energy and perseverance was required to produce a small stream of sparkling cold water.

The kitchen itself was a nice bright room with three long horizontal windows with frilly white curtains. The walls and ceiling were freshly painted a light beige. A set of table and chairs completed the furnishings.

Turning back towards the hall, one could see a closed door to the right. "This is the patient's room," said the nurse as she opened it and waited for me to enter. "We have had only one patient during the past year, so we are using it now as a cool room for our food. Our supply of ice has run out, so by keeping the blind drawn and the door closed it stays quite cool." Besides a hospital bed covered with a white spread, the room contained a serviceable washstand made of wooden packing boxes covered with a sheet, holding an enamelled wash basin and pitcher, soap dish and other such necessities. Against the wall were more packing boxes or orange crates stacked on end, serving as a cupboard for food.

To the left of the hall, an archway opened into a similar room, but this one was cluttered with a large cupboard filled with blankets and other linens, and with innumerable boxes and bundles of supplies and medicines. Fortunately, heavy green drapes hid this display from the living room.

We climbed the steep narrow stairs and I was surprised to find three large bright bedrooms and a storeroom. I was told that the year before a building firm in the city [8] had very kindly donated sufficient gyproc to cover all walls and ceilings upstairs and that someone else contributed the paint. No wonder these rooms looked so much nicer than those downstairs.

The bedrooms were all furnished with old hospital beds with thin hard mattresses. Two had chintz-covered boxes for dressers and wash stands but, in the nurse's room, they were real, although by no means elaborate. When I looked out of her window I knew that this was going to be my room as soon as she moved out, for at the end of the long back yard was a real lake! Imagine me, a city gal living on a lake!

The nurse, perhaps for reasons of her own, avoided mentioning the heating system or the "basement." I would learn about them later, the hard way. Well, so much for the building. Not much like a hospital, but I could see its possibilities and it was mine. I would make a hospital of it.

Next on the tour was the backyard. It was very large compared to the city lots of my experience. A woodpile extended along the fence on the left side and ended at the "phone booth"[9] (no indoor plumbing here) about a third of the way down the yard. From there on down to the shaky-looking building at the end was junk: old lumber, posts, and packing boxes. The nurse said it was mostly the remains of the old shed torn down to make room for the new kitchen.

A steep bank sloped down to the shore, which looked to me like a good beach. I was told that the fishing was very good, especially for black bass and mud cats. The end building mentioned extended out over the bank and the part underneath was used for storing ice. Large blocks were cut out on the lake during the winter, drawn in and packed in sawdust for use during the summer. The upper part of the building was used as a garage where the nurse kept her car. It didn't look very safe to me. While a small patch of lawn and flowerbed near the house helped to brighten the yard, the rest was a wild confusion of weeds.

The nurse suggested we go for a short walk up the road. It was then that I learned why each lot was fenced in and the gates closed. Nearly every family in the village kept a cow or two, she told me, and here they were, milling all around. Some were even lying in the middle of the road. They grazed in the fields and woods during the day but, after the evening milking, they were generally left to spend the night close to home to be handy for the early morning milking. And woe betide anyone who had a garden and neglected to keep his gate tightly shut! I was told later about one cow that discovered she could open several of the gates by a slight twist of her horn on the latch. And I soon learned that if I had to walk through town after dark it was wise to carry a light. During the day the road was always clean, as one of the neighbours went out with his shovel and wheelbarrow early every morning and gathered up all the manure. He always had a well-fertilized garden.

As we walked up the road we passed a plain little white church[10] and a fairly large red brick school. Its size surprised me, but the nurse told me that it was a two-room Consolidated Continuation School, which meant that it had been built to accommodate the children from more than one school section and that the first two years of high school were taught there.[11]

We followed the road as it curved sharply to the right at the foot of a steep hill. Soon we could see the most beautiful view, one which actually brought tears to my eyes. As the nurse had planned to spend the evening with friends, we soon returned to the Outpost. There, Aileen and I had the chance to become better acquainted. We were going to live together so were naturally anxious to learn a bit about each other.

As twilight was setting in, Aileen lit the little coal oil lamp and put it on its high shelf in the hall, with the reflector behind it. I had been introduced to this wonderful invention as a child when visiting my grandparents on the farm but had never been required to handle one myself. Now, however, I would no doubt have to know how to operate such lamps, therefore I very attentively watched her every movement. With the hall light in place, she proceeded to light a tall one which, she said, she would leave on the kitchen table. Then she said, "Now, I'll show you how to light the Coleman." She did!

The Coleman lamp burned gasoline. It had a large round base holding the fuel, from the centre of which ran a long tube with two white bag-like affairs at the top. These were mantles, she said, which produced the light. A large white opaque glass shade fitted on a frame over these and a long rod on top was to hang it from a hook in the ceiling. There were two screw caps in the top of the base, one of which opened for filling. That had been done in the morning. Aileen unscrewed the other, then, using a small tube-like pump, she pumped and pumped to fill it with air which would force the fuel to the top. That part seemed fine, but when she held a lighted match to it, flames shot up, I was sure, to the ceiling! I expected an explosion, but she laughed and said it was just warming up. In a short time the lamp settled down. Aileen opened the valve and a clear white light came on, every bit as bright as an electric bulb. Many a dark night passed, however, before I had the courage to put into practice what I had learned that night! If the Outpost were to go up in flames, it certainly would not be by my hands!

Finally, we settled down to have a cozy little chat, Aileen with her embroidery and I with some knitting. Evidently she had been worrying as to whether or not I would keep her on as housekeeper. Perhaps I would rather have an older person. She was a local girl of 15 and had been working at the Outpost for almost a year. She looked on it as her [second] home.[12] I assured her that I had no intention of making a change as long as we could get along together satisfactorily.

"Will you do the cooking?" she asked.

"Oh, no indeed," I said, "I don't expect to have time to do anything like that." (Besides, I really didn't want her to know how little I knew of that art.) "Don't you do the cooking now?" I asked.

"No, Nurse does all of that. I don't know much about cooking. I just wash the dishes and keep the house clean."

"Do you think you could learn?" I asked.

"I would sure like to if you are willing to take a chance."

"I'm not afraid," I replied, "And I'm sure we'll get along fine." So, with that problem settled to our mutual satisfaction, we went on to discuss her other duties.

"I will give you complete charge of the housekeeping," I told her. "Do you think you could manage that?"

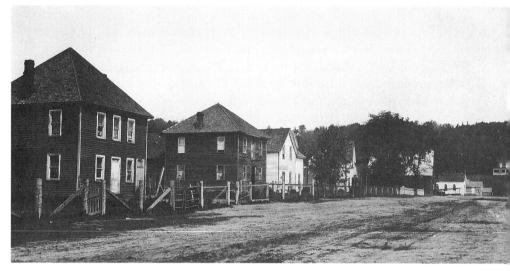

A view of the buildings on the west side of the main part of Wilberforce, circa 1930s. In sequence from front left: the Charles Bowen home; the George Miller (later to become Gertrude's father-in-law) home; White's Boarding House; Ames' house; the Orange Hall; St. Margaret's Anglican Church; and the Wilberforce School. The house on the hill may have been owned by Mrs. Fowlie at this time. *Courtesy Wilberforce Heritage Guild Collection.*

"Oh, I'd love to try!" She seemed delighted. "I'll do my very best," she said enthusiastically. She seemed such an intelligent girl for her age, and I felt that she might thrive on such a responsibility. I was right. From that evening on, I had no reason whatsoever to be concerned about any part of the housekeeping. Before long she was one of the best cooks in the community, and that is really saying something. As to her housekeeping ability and her role as a companion, well, she was a jewel. She also helped greatly with the nursing when I was in need of extra hands.

That first evening was a fine start for both Aileen and myself. She was very reassuring, telling me how little work the nurse had been required to do this past year, not even any emergencies.

This was Wednesday and, as I would not be officially on duty until Saturday evening, the next three days were well filled and passed very quickly. The nurse and I spent the first morning going over books, records, supplies and the work in general. There was so much I wanted to know about my duties and once more I was told that there really was not much to be done except to go when sent for. First, and most important to me, was where could the nearest doctor be reached

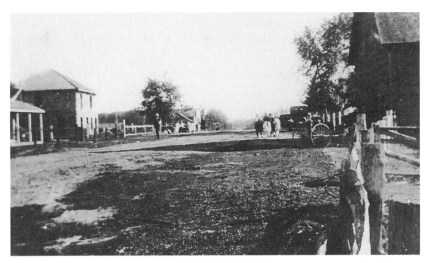

The postcard shows the main street, looking south. The large clapboard building with the buggy in front is the Orange Hall. On the left is the verandah of Charles McMahon's house and Marshall's stone house, the post office. The buildings, left, in the distance are stores. Circa 1920s. *Courtesy Wilberforce Heritage Guild Collection.*

and how could I get in touch with him, since there was no telephone at the Outpost. My heart almost stopped when she told me, "There are two doctors in Haliburton, about 25 miles from here, and one in Bancroft, about 30 miles in the other direction."

The road to Bancroft, she said, was much worse than the road to Haliburton, but Bancroft was on the I.B.&O. Railway,[13] so it was easier to get a doctor from there during the winter when roads were blocked with snow.

"How can I get in touch with a doctor in case of an emergency?" I asked. "And what about confinements?" Well, I learned that there was one telephone in the village and it was located in the store. It was a railway telephone, connecting the stations along the line. As there was no station agent, Mr. Agnew,[14] the storekeeper, was the acting agent, looking after freight and other goods. So the telephone was there. When a doctor was needed, he would call the Gooderham station and have their people relay the message over another line to the doctor in Haliburton. Or he would call the Bancroft station and the message would be relayed to the doctor there. I must have looked upset at this information, for the nurse hastened to assure me that there really wasn't anything to worry about as Mr. Agnew was very understanding and most kind in looking after messages. Anyway, it was very seldom that any such need arose.

15

That afternoon we visited a few homes in the village, walking down one side of the road and up the other. We skipped the first house where Mr. and Mrs. Charlie McMahon and two of their sons lived, and our first call was at the Marshalls' who kept the Post Office in part of their big stone house. Mr. Tom Marshall was a war amputee and he and his wife[15] made a jolly pair. They had quite a large family. Next was the general store owned by Mr. and Mrs. Fred Agnew. Their home adjoined the store and they had two boys, Ross and Murray.

The road led down the hill to the railroad but directly opposite the store was the home of Mr. and Mrs. George Webber and their adult daughter, "Bert."[16] They were retired farmers. The next building was vacant, "being used as a hall," I was told. The people living in the adjacent house were a retired English couple, Mr. and Mrs. A.W. [Alfred] Fleming and their son Leonard, a real English gentleman. Their next-door neighbours were the Bowen family, Mr. and Mrs. Charlie Bowen and their five children.[17] Then came the home of George Miller.[18] George had two boys still at school, one daughter married, one attending Normal School in North Bay, and an older son working at a sawmill elsewhere in the county.

The big white building beside the Millers was the boarding house, a place of constant activity, interest and fun. It was run by Mrs. Sid White,[19] who had taken it over from her mother,[20] a woman now in her 80s but still full of wit and wisdom. The two teachers boarded there as well as Miss Taylor,[21] the Deaconess, who very ably attended to the spiritual needs of the community. This house was also the stopping place for salesmen, lumber scalers and other travellers in town for short periods. Directly across from the Outpost was the Orange Hall,[22] a large barn-like structure, yet a place of many important activities.

Everyone was so friendly and the time passed so quickly that we had to leave the rest until a later date. No longer did I feel like a stranger in a strange land.

The next afternoon we went to Haliburton so that I might meet the doctors there. I shall never forget that trip! The road! Nothing but hills, rocks and curves, twenty-five miles of them! Those poor doctors! What if I should need one in a hurry? I was certainly glad not to be doing the driving, otherwise I could not have enjoyed the gorgeous scenery. We would just nicely reach the bottom of one hill when there would be either a sharp turn or another hill, or possibly both. Sometimes a sharp curve would appear part way up or down a hill. One series of ups and downs and twists was known as "Vinegar Hill." Later I was told that a farmer who lived at the very top many years ago had named it. He had driven his team and wagon to Haliburton one fall to get his winter supply of food and other necessities which included a barrel of vinegar. Just as he reached the top of the hill, a wheel came off the wagon, causing the barrel to roll off and right on down to the bottom of the hill, spilling vinegar all the way.

After about two hours,[23] we arrived at the top of another steep hill and stopped. "It will be a few minutes until we reach Haliburton," said the nurse, "But if you look to the right through those trees, you can see it." This spot was "Dover's Hill," and there far below, nestled around one side of a small lake, was the village. We followed the winding road down the steep incline, with me holding my breath and hoping the brakes were good. Finally, we stopped in front of the impressive home and office of Dr. [John] Speck.

After spending a delightful half-hour or so with the doctor and his wife, we went on up the street to Dr. [Charles E.] Frain's office. He was busy at the time so asked us to go to his home. He would follow shortly. Once again we enjoyed our visit and when the doctor arrived, his wife served tea and cookies. Soon we left for our return journey home. Both doctors had been very friendly and assured me that they would be very happy to work with me and would help whenever I needed them. It had been a very profitable afternoon for me, for now I felt that I was not entirely alone in this work, even though the doctors were so far away.

That night I was introduced to my first country dance at Gooderham. Although I suffered a few embarrassing moments, the experience was immensely enjoyable. I certainly met a lot of people and acquired an insight into the social life of this community. Amazingly, I struggled through several square dances without much difficulty. Fortunately, everyone was there for fun so were not too critical. There were two things which impressed me most about the evening. Firstly, I was amazed at the large number of children of all ages that were there. No baby-sitters in those days! Before the evening was over, the platform floor appeared to be a giant bed with little children stretched out all over it, sound asleep. Secondly, the amount of sandwiches, cakes and tea that were served and consumed about midnight was incredible. It was in the wee small hours when we returned to the Outpost. What a life! Would it continue like this?

We spent Saturday afternoon calling at a few farmhouses within a couple miles of the village. One in particular interested me: the home, a log house, belonging to Mrs. Earle,[24] a widow with two teenage sons. They lived at the foot of a long steep hill. The boys, Stephen and George, attended school in town and, with their mother's help, were carrying on the work of the farm. They were full of fun and mischief so there was never a dull moment. Mrs. Earle, a jolly little English woman, insisted on us staying long enough to have a cup of tea and a piece of cake. She said she would like to read my cup[25] and see what was in store for me. And, of course, I was all for wanting to know too. She said that according to my cup, my stay here would be long and happy, though I would be kept very busy. Never were truer words spoken, for I spent forty-four happy busy years in the community.

Before supper that evening, the nurse bade us farewell and about the same time my knees began to shake. I was now on twenty-four hour duty, seven days a week, and twenty-five miles from a doctor!

2

Meet the Challenge:
Hit the Floor Running

Well, this was Saturday evening. I had spent three wonderful days in this peaceful little village. I could call them holidays, for there hadn't been a hint of work done. And from all reports, this is the way it would likely continue, far different from the activities at the hospital back home. There, we would be on the wards at 7 a.m. rushing about, carrying bed pans, giving treatments, bathing patients, and with nothing more interesting to see than plain white walls.

My predecessor, who had so kindly introduced me to my neighbours and everything in general, had departed.[1] From now on I would be completely on my own in this large wilderness. Little did I dream that before long I would be known not only as "The Nurse," but midwife, doctor, undertaker, social worker, as well as family counsellor. But, as they say, "Ignorance is bliss." I wasn't worrying. Mrs. Earle's glimpse into the future had been forgotten and I hadn't even bothered to unpack my trunk. I would have plenty of time for that later. But little did I know about the habits of "Mr. Stork" in this country!

Before daylight Sunday morning, I was awakened by the tinkling sound of a bell. I opened my eyes to find my room almost in darkness except for a faint grayness at the window. I felt for my flashlight, then waited to make sure I hadn't been dreaming. There it was again, a

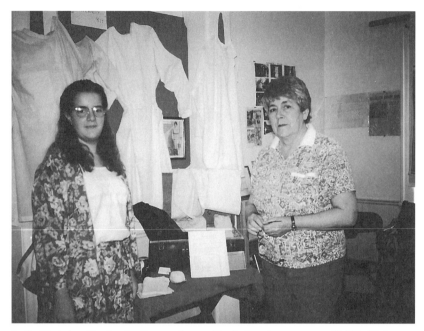

Left, Christine Hattin, the first student guide during the summer of 1993. Right, Hilda Clark, President of the Wilberforce Heritage Guild at that time. The display in the background features the nurse's "black bag," the maternity kit. *Courtesy Wilberforce Heritage Guild Collection.*

rasping sound and a little tinkle. Something will certainly have to be done about that bell, I thought. I slipped into my dressing gown and slippers and, with flashlight in hand, hurried down the stairs and opened the door. There stood a tall young man who, without ceremony, said, "Mrs. E.[2] needs you right away!"

I recalled that the nurse had mentioned that a Mrs. E. was expecting in two or three weeks. This must be the one. "Is she…," I started to ask, but before I could say any more, he blurted out, "Yes, yes I think so! I'll wait in the car." I told him I would hurry. Rushing back to my room, I found that Aileen, bless her, had lit my lamp. Where should I start? Instead of running around making social calls, going to dances and relying on the assurance of the nurse that there was hardly any calls, why hadn't I spent my time getting things in order for what "might happen." After all, that's why I was here. Well, that was lesson number one.

I had trained in an up-to-date, well equipped hospital where a baby was seldom born with less than one doctor and two or three nurses

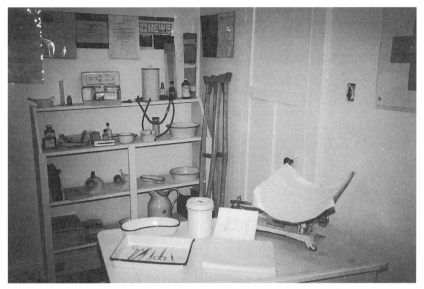

The Nurse's Office in the Outpost Museum, displaying original artifacts including the baby scales. *Courtesy Wilberforce Heritage Guild Collection.*

in attendance. A table would be located with sterile supplies, basins, instruments, dressings, sheets, all the attendant needs. Dismissing those thoughts, I hurriedly donned my uniform and picked up my equipment, a large suitcase[3] which the nurse had shown me, saying that it was always kept in readiness, "just in case." This contained everything that would be needed (almost), such as rubber sheet, sterile sheets, dressings, gowns, basins, baby clothes, and so on. And, of course, I also took the black bag which always accompanied the nurse on her visits. Inside were the simple medicines, instruments, and first aid equipment. This bag, too, was always kept in readiness.

I breathed a little prayer for the guidance, thankful for my month with the V.O.N.,[4] and I was ready. Climbing into the ancient Model T, I sat beside the chap who'd been waiting, and we were on our way. I wondered if this man was the patient's husband or perhaps a neighbour. He didn't seem to want to talk and, once we were on our way, I had no desire to take his mind off his driving.

To travel leisurely through this hilly country in broad daylight was one thing, but to rattle downhill at breath-taking speed and to race around hairpin curves in a Model T at break of dawn was a different matter. I realize now that we couldn't have been travelling more than 20 miles an hour, but to me, glimpsing walls of rock through the mist

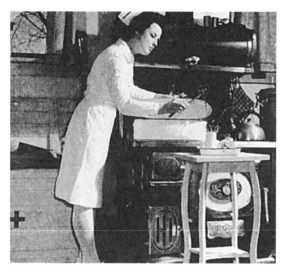

Dorothy Stoughton (Mrs. Floyd Short), house-keeper at the Outpost in 1940s, poses in nurse's uniform to illustrate the sterilizer being used on the kitchen cookstove, sterilizing instruments. Note the huge woodbox with the Red Cross on it. *Courtesy Wilberforce Guild Collection, donated by a former resident, Mrs. Alice Sedgwick.*

as we followed the narrow rough road, we seemed to be breaking all speed records. I was trying my best to keep my mind on the patient, while hanging on for dear life, and wishing the nurse had taken me to see her. Perhaps it was because of the road, one that was much worse than any we had ever travelled on together.

Several times I was about to ask the driver a question, but decided it would be far better for me to reach the patient in complete ignorance of the situation than not to arrive at all. I just hung on and prayed that everything would be all right. At one point, however, I did get up enough courage to ask how far we had to go, and was told about five miles. By the time we had chugged up the last hill, (and what hill! I was terrified that the car wouldn't make it), it was quite light. There, nestled in a little hollow at the very top of the hill, was a weather-beaten house overlooking a beautiful little lake far, far below. I could see for miles! But this was no time to be admiring the view.

I hurried up to the door and was met by a frail old lady in a big white apron. "Hurry, Nurse," she said, as she led me through a couple of rooms. But before we reached the bedroom door, I heard a baby's healthy cry! My first case and the stork had beaten me! He must have passed us on that last hill! However, there was still plenty for me to do, though the patient's mother had everything pretty well under control. She told me later that she had attended many of her neighbours at childbirth before the Outpost had been opened. She had managed things quite well here, and everything was clean, which wasn't always

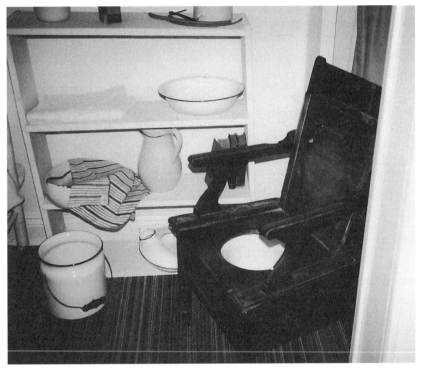

A view of one end of the patient's room as displayed in the Outpost Museum.
Courtesy Wilberforce Heritage Guild Collection.

the case in other homes, as I was to learn later.

I took care of mother and baby and before long the mother was resting comfortably and the baby girl[5] bathed and asleep. I was then called to the kitchen for breakfast. Breakfast! What a table! When I saw it I thought surely they must have been combining all the meals of the day. Fried potatoes, fried pork, homemade bread, slices at least an inch thick and nearly a foot across, homemade butter, preserves, pie, a big three-layer cake and a big jug of milk. Needless to say, I wasn't able to partake of everything in spite of the coaxing, but I certainly did relish the meal.

When I thought it would be quite safe to leave the patient, I informed my chauffeur, who, incidentally, turned out to be the patient's brother. We started off. This time he didn't drive nearly so fast and was a great deal more talkative. He informed me that he had put a lot of work on the car since morning, then asked, "What would you have said this morning if you had known that there were no brakes on the car?" No wonder he didn't feel like talking!

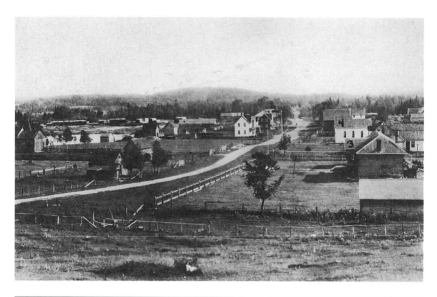

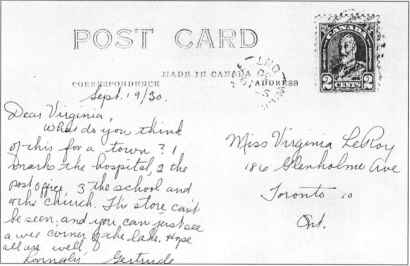

This postcard was purchased at Agnew's General Store in Wilberforce. During Gertrude LeRoy's first month at the Outpost, she sent this card home to her sister in Toronto. She even numbered the buildings! *Courtesy Gloria (Luckock) Wigg, niece of Gertrude LeRoy Miller.*

It was almost noon when we arrived in town. My first day on duty and my first confinement over and without a doctor! Did this mean that I was going to have a busy time here? Perhaps Mrs. Earle was right after all. Well, at least I was learning that I could make myself useful in this community. I certainly did not want it to be a life of leisure as had been described.

Most of the afternoon was spent cleaning up and repacking the big suitcase, just in case. The linens were put to soak, utensils washed, wrapped, and sterilized, along with clean sheets, and other amenities. The sterilizing was done in a large pressure cooker on the kitchen stove. A covered granite dish was used for boiling instruments as needed at the Outpost.

After the unexpected call on Sunday, I began to wonder what I would do if an emergency case were brought in. The patient's room was being used as a pantry and the other downstairs room was cluttered with supplies and cupboards stuffed with goods, all of which I thought should be upstairs in the storeroom. I decided that I must have a suitable place to interview patients, do dressings, give treatments and keep records. Also, there must be a room ready to accommodate a patient on a moment's notice. This was my hospital now and I intended to see that it was a real nice one.

On Monday, Aileen rounded up a couple of husky fellows who pitched in and carried the big linen cupboard and other heavy things upstairs, then moved the big desk in from the living room. I set up a washstand with basin, brushes, green soap and a large pitcher of water. Soon the room resembled a real hospital office and treatment centre. The downstairs patient's room was re-arranged and made ready for business.

The next few days passed so quickly. I had been told that none of my predecessors had had any training in Public Health Nursing, so it was up to me to set up a Public Health program. What a challenge! Where should I begin? There should be more health teaching in the schools, along with immunization of all school and preschool children, as well as of adults, against diphtheria and smallpox. Diphtheria toxoid was new and had not yet been introduced in this area so I would have to get the idea of immunization across to all parents. Also, I wanted to start Baby Clinics and Home Nursing classes. I could hardly wait to get started.

The map of Haliburton County, which I had dug up and hung on the office wall, was studied with care. Aileen, who was a wonderful source of information, helped me locate the schools and villages that I was expected to serve; all of the schools in Monmouth Township as well as some in the surrounding townships, twelve schools in all. They were: Wilberforce (2 rooms), Tory Hill, Hotspur, Hadlington, Essonville, Bear

Lake, Cheddar, Harcourt, Highland Grove North, Highland Grove South, Kennaway and Beech Ridge.

I was shocked to discover that some were nearly twenty miles away, and only accessible over those windy, rugged roads! For the first time I realized the significance of this job I had undertaken. The health of the inhabitants of this tremendous territory was more or less dependent on me! One thing I knew for sure, I couldn't handle it alone, but with God's help I could and would!

The important thing, I decided, was to make a plan, and stick to it in order that every part of the area would be served as equitably as possible. It wasn't very long, however, until I learned lesson number two; plans are very necessary, but to follow them to the letter when the human element is involved is both impossible and impractical.

As soon as things were fairly well organized at the Outpost, I decided to call on the other known pre-natal patient. Hence, I set out to find her. I was to go up the road, then follow an old road. My patient lived in the first house I would encounter.

"It will be very rough walking," Aileen warned, "So don't wear high heels." And rough it was! It might have been a road at one time, but it certainly couldn't be called one now with all the deep ruts and rocks. Weeds, brush and even small trees pretty well covered the area from fence to fence.

As I climbed the hill I looked back; I was thrilled with the view. The sky was clear blue with fleecy white clouds drifting above the layers of green and yellow hills. Here and there the hills were enriched by touches of orange and red, pierced frequently by the dark spikes of evergreens. What an awesome sight! Here I was, a part of this beautiful creation, a tool in the hands of my Maker, sent to care for the sick and to promote health throughout this exceptional land. The prayers, which I formed in my mind, could not be put into words, but I knew I was not alone.

Onward I trudged, the path becoming rougher and rougher, with berry and bramble bushes crowding in on either side. Finally, I came to a clearing. I heard a dog bark and decided I must be nearing my destination. Soon an old weather-worn two-story house, quite in keeping with the old sheds and broken-down fences of its surroundings, came into view. A little patch of garden with a few bright flowers was the only sign that there was someone here who cared.

Before I could reach the house two little tots appeared, seemingly from nowhere, and ran into the house. Their mother appeared at the door. She was pitifully thin and worn out, looking very pregnant. "Hello," I called, "Are you Mrs. M.?"

"Yes," she answered, smiling. I could see that she was pleased to have a visitor.

"I'm Miss LeRoy, the new nurse," I informed her. "It is such a nice day I thought I'd come see you."

"I'm glad you came, Nurse. Come in."

As I followed her into the house I didn't have to be told that this was a real poverty-stricken home, but a clean home. Just the bare essentials were in this large room. The two children were very shy at first, but later played on the floor with two little puppies.

"That's quite a walk up here," I said, trying to start a conversation. "I suppose you don't get to the village very often."

"No, I don't, and not many come here either," she said. "But Tom goes to town everyday. He does a bit of work here and there. I'm glad you came to see me. I suppose the other nurse told you I'd be calling you before long."

"Yes, but she didn't give me much information to go on. I know you have other children, is it five?"

"Well, there's five living, but I've had a lot more than that. I've sort of lost track but I think this will be my thirteenth." Seven had died! No doubt they had all died of malnutrition. She certainly looked as if she could stand a few good meals, though she said she was feeling quite well.

As this was my first pre-natal visit here, I followed the regular V.O.N. routine regarding questions and recording information. Her answers were so shocking that my heart ached for her. All of her twelve children had been born at home, wherever that happened to be at the time. (I learned later that they were squatters and moved frequently). Not once had a doctor attended her. Sometimes she had been lucky and her husband had gone for the nurse, otherwise a neighbour, or whoever happened to be handy, attended to her. And after-care? Well, it was a natural function so why all the fuss? It was no wonder the poor woman looked so tired and worn out. If I could only persuade her to come to the Outpost this time. There she would have a complete rest, good meals and proper care, and the new baby would get a good start in life, at least for ten days. Those were the days when a mother MUST stay in bed for ten days after giving birth.

"How would you like to have this baby at the Outpost, Mrs. M.?" I asked. "It would give you a chance to have a good rest and I could look after you so much better there."

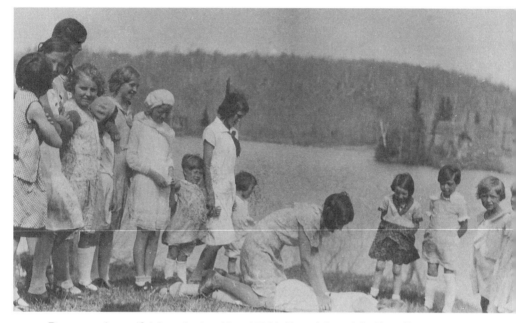

Demonstrating artificial respiration (circa 1930s). From left to right: Irma Bowen, Kay Fleming, _____, Helen Marshall, _____, Aileen Fleming, Thelma Greer (?), Edith Tallman (giving respiration), Winnie Fleming, _____. Dark Lake is in the background. *Courtesy Wilberforce Heritage Guild Collection, donated by Aileen Ames Walker.*

"It would be nice alright, but there wouldn't be anyone here to get meals and look after the children."

"What about your husband? He is around most of the time isn't he? Perhaps he could plan to stay around, and Susie must be old enough to help a bit after school."

"Well, I don't know what Tom will say to it, but I'll tell him what you said," she replied.

"You say you still have about three more weeks to go, so just try to take it easy. I'll be back to see you in a few days."

The trip back to the Outpost didn't seem to take as nearly so long but it did give me some time to do some thinking. What an out-of-the-way-place for a woman in Mrs. M.'s condition. No doubt I'd run across similar situations in the future. This was merely my first problem. I wondered what had given my predecessor the idea that there was no work to be done in this community. There were twelve schools to be visited. What about the homes of all those school children? There must be many infants and pre-school children as well as mothers in those homes who could be helped along the road to good health. Wasn't that the reason the Outpost had been started in the first place? Of course, previous nurses had not had Public Health training.

At present my problem was Mrs. M. Anyone could see that she would need more than a few minutes of nursing care after her baby arrives. If we had her at the Outpost for ten days, a few wholesome meals would do wonders for her as well as the baby, not to mention the rest she would have.

Fortunately, the Red Cross Committee was to meet very soon. This committee was made up of members of the local Red Cross Branch and was responsible for the building, fuel and general upkeep of the Outpost. The Ontario Division provided the Nursing Service, medical supplies and food. Whatever fees were collected, which incidentally amounted to very little in those days, they were sent to Red Cross Headquarters. Usually, any interested local resident was welcome to attend these meetings and often many did.

I had received a letter from Headquarters informing me that Miss Hamilton would arrive on Wednesday and wished to meet with the Committee on Thursday evening. I was delighted, for now I could get official advice regarding the "M" situation from both the local committee and Headquarters. I was anxious, too, for Miss Hamilton to see what I had been doing. Aileen immediately began planning the lunch she would serve, a very important part of every such meeting.

Before train time Wednesday, everything was in readiness to welcome our guest. The exact arrival time was always unpredictable, but as Mr. Agnew kept in touch by telephone with the stations along the line, he could tell us the approximate expected time. Thus, Aileen could start the dinner and I could be at the station to meet the train. As I had learned earlier, meeting the train was a favourite pastime of many of the villagers for, after all, how else could they keep in touch with the outside world? As a rule there would be a passenger or two that someone knew and who could exchange the latest news from along the line while the freight was being unloaded, box cars picked up and passengers exchanged. It was really surprising how much gossip could be gleaned in thirty minutes.

We spent Wednesday evening and most of Thursday going over the work in general. I had so many questions to ask Miss Hamilton. She seemed pleased with my accomplishments to date and also my plans for the future, and offered many helpful suggestions. Regarding the "M" matter, she felt as I did concerning the need but suggested we let the Committee decide whether or not to bring the patient to the Outpost.

The Thursday meeting was well attended and very long, due to the fact that many of the people seldom had an opportunity to spend an evening together, especially those living outside the village. The farmers had to discuss their problems, and compare prices they were getting for eggs, wool and beef with those of a few years ago. However, a surprising amount of Outpost business was transacted as well.

I learned that the Committee (in other words, The Monmouth Charitable Association,[6] the name under which the Charter was held) had a large debt on its shoulders. Not only was the building still not completely paid for, but wood must be provided for the winter and several repairs were badly needed. It was decided to hold a Masquerade Dance at Halloween to raise funds to carry on the service. I was appointed to act on that committee.

Finally, I brought up the matter of admitting Mrs. M. This family was well known to everyone and the mere mention of the name was like touching a lighted match to a pile of dry leaves. Nearly everyone had a little story to tell about Tom and his escapades, all very enlightening to me. Tom, it seemed, was a very good worker, when he felt like working, which wasn't too often. Everyone felt sorry for his wife.

I explained that after a woman has had several children, her muscles sometimes lose their elasticity and complications could develop. It would be a great help to have her at the Outpost in case something did go wrong.

I realized that Tom would make no effort to pay anything towards his wife's care. I'd been told that he had never been known to pay for any previous services. On the other hand, the Outpost was there for a purpose. It had been open for over eight years and so far only nine babies had been born in it.[7] Why not put it to better use? Both mother and baby would have constant care and a chance to get built up. And so it was unanimously agreed that I should try to persuade Mrs. M. to come to the Outpost to have her baby. Incidentally, the daily rates for hospital care at that time were $1.50 for the mother and $0.50 for the baby.

After I helped Aileen serve the tasty lunch she had prepared, the pleasant and encouraging evening was over. I was really very lucky, I decided, to be working in such a pleasant atmosphere.

Before leaving Friday morning, Miss Hamilton told me that she felt I was quite capable of carrying on the work and that I was not to hes-

These receipts confirm that the rates mentioned by author were still the same in 1932, two years later. *Courtesy Wilberforce Heritage Guild Collection.*

itate about asking for advice or help from the office. My courage was considerably strengthened by her visit.

To my great relief, Mrs. M. decided to come to the Outpost. The evening before she was due to have her baby, Aileen and I went for her. We had assured her that there was no need to bring anything as there were hospital gowns available and the neighbours had made up an ample layette.

It was such a thrill for us to admit a patient. The atmosphere of the whole building was changed and we were in business as a hospital. The "pantry" had been transformed into an immaculate hospital room, which would require only a few minutes to convert into a delivery room. That evening Mrs. M. was very quiet, no doubt worrying about her children, though she said she was sure they would be all right.

Nothing happened during the night, but the patient was up and dressed bright and early the next morning. "I think, Nurse," she said, "I'll just go home and see how things are. I'll come back this evening, unless I have to come back sooner."

Would she come back? Perhaps she needed the assurance that everything was fine at home. So, after a good breakfast, we set out. I decided to accompany her in case the exertion of the long walk might bring on labour, and was surprised when she seemed to stand the trip as well as I did. I had forgotten that in spite of her condition she was used to far more hard work than I was.

We were both relieved to find things quite normal at home. The older children had gone to school, Tom had actually washed the breakfast dishes, and he and the two little ones were about to come see their mother. I thought they looked a little disappointed at being deprived of the rare outing. The mother insisted on staying and her husband said he would see that she got back safely.

This procedure was repeated for the next two days. At least she was getting exercise, a hearty breakfast every morning and a bedtime snack at night. These factors, even for that short time, should be helpful. She had told me that there had never been any complications, but after so many pregnancies I was not looking forward to delivering her by myself. I had notified Dr. Frain about her case and he suggested that I go ahead, but if I suspected any trouble to call him.

About the middle of the fourth night, her bell signalled me to get on the job. Within an hour we had a wee baby girl after a normal delivery. This was quite an experience for me, my first complete delivery without a doctor. I had sincerely hoped that the need to contend with complications would not arise.

I am quite sure that no mother or baby ever received better care and attention than these two did during the next ten days. Mrs. M. was a perfect patient, the only problem being to keep her in bed. The dainty trays Aileen carried in to her would tempt the poorest appetite, but this patient needed no tempting. I am sure she gained weight and this was the first real rest she had ever had in her life. Her baby gained steadily and was named after Aileen and myself.

At first, Tom came everyday to visit his wife and sat with her for an hour or so. It was really my fault that he didn't come back after about the sixth day. We were having trouble with our pump,[8] and with so much extra laundry to be done, we needed a great deal of water. From all reports, I had understood that Tom was a real handyman and could do a good job at anything if he really wanted to. So this day, while he was visiting his wife, I explained our situation and asked if he would mind trying to fix the pump. He jumped up, "Sorry, Nurse," he said, "I have a job waiting for me up the road. If you can't get anyone else, I'll have a look at it tomorrow." That was last we saw of Tom while his wife was with us. When she was ready to go home, one of the neighbours brought his team and wagon and braved the old road to her home. It must have been a very rough ride, but far better for her than walking.

Several times while she was at the Outpost, I left mother and baby in Aileen's care while I ventured out to nearby schools. By the end of October, I had visited all twelve. Now, better equipped with an under-standing of what went on in the various areas and what some of the school needs were, I could make plans accordingly.

3

Dealing With Loneliness

The summer season was over when I arrived in Wilberforce and it took me a little while to become oriented to this new environ-ment. However, it wasn't long until I realized that my participation in the social activites of the community was as important to the people here as my professional duties. After all, if I wanted any social life this is where I would have to find it. There could be no weekend trips to the city.

Miss Annie Taylor, the [Anglican] Deaconess, was a real friend in the wilderness. She had received a little training in nursing (also at T.W.H.[1]) and offered to help out any time, but I would not dream of asking her to take over any responsibility. Actually, I never felt bored or lonely. Aileen was good company and knew everyone, so we often made social calls together. It was such a good way to get to know the people and, even without telephones, the whole neighborhood always seemed to know where to find me if I was needed. The two teachers, Marjory Chambers and Ed Edmonds, were very good company as well.

I had never been greatly interested in playing cards, but I soon learned that if I wished to be a member of Wilberforce society I would have to learn to play euchre. A short time after my arrival there was to be a euchre party at Beech Ridge School, about four miles away. Everyone was welcome. It had been arranged by the teacher, Miss Kay

Crosson, to raise money to buy something for the school. Several Wilberforce people were going and the Marshalls kindly invited me to go with them. At this time I had not yet visited this school, so most of the people as well as the teacher were strangers to me. I was surprised to see so many children there with their parents. It seemed that parents took their children to card parties as well as dances, which of course was much better than leaving them home alone.

The desks were piled along one wall and the room was filled with small tables and chairs. The children who were old enough were at tables on the platform, playing games of their own such as checkers and crokinole, while the very small ones were on their parents' laps at the card tables. I was quite shocked to see one mother nursing her baby while playing. No one appeared to notice anything wrong, so I decided this must just be one of the things I would have to get used to in my new home.

It was progressive euchre and I didn't do very well at first. When at last I did catch on, it was too late and I was given the "Booby" prize! To me that was as thrilling as if I'd won first prize, but the teacher seemed to be awfully embarrassed when she presented it to me. It was not until I opened the neatly wrapped parcel bearing the tag saying, "Something for your neck," that I realized why. It was a cake of Lux Toilet Soap! That little incident really broke the ice for me in that community.

One evening about two weeks after my arrival, Aileen and her friends, Ethel and Neoma Marshall, were having an exciting discussion in our kitchen. After awhile they called me in. "This town has been so dead lately," said Ethel. "We've decided to get up a dance for Saturday night. Some of the boys will be home from camp and we're sure we know where we can get someone to play.[2] What do you think of the idea?"

"It sounds good to me," I answered. "But where will you have it?"

"We can have it at the Orange Hall, across the road." Having attended the one dance in Gooderham, I figured that it would be mostly square dance.

"I'm not a square dancer," I continued. "But it's fun to watch. Anyway, I won't have a partner."

"That doesn't matter," said Ethel. "We'll all go together, and likely all the men will want to dance with the new nurse."

"Too bad Del Miller isn't around," piped up Aileen. "I'm sure he would be the first man to ask you to dance."

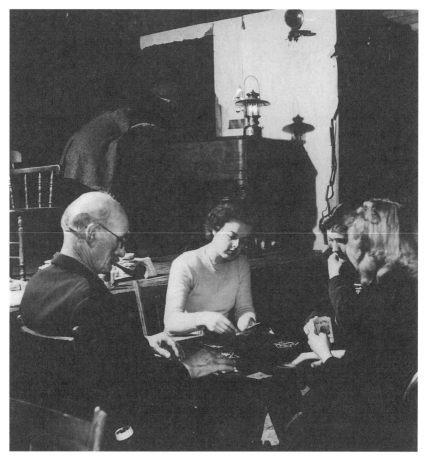

The Orange Hall was used for many activities—everything from dances to Christmas concerts to playing cards. Here, playing euchre are (left to right): Fred Barnes, Dorothy (Stoughton) Short and Edith (Tallman) Daniels, circa 1946. Note the raised stage and the coleman lamp placed on the piano to provide some of the light. *Courtesy Wilberforce Heritage Guild Collection, donated by Red Cross Headquarters, Ottawa.*

I was curious. "Who is Del Miller and why isn't he around?"

"He is away working at a sawmill, but some weekends he comes home. You just watch! The first time he's home, he'll find an excuse to meet you," Aileen conjectured. "I think you will like him. He's tall, dark and handsome."

"Well, here's hoping he comes in time for the dance."

The girls went ahead with their plans and before long everyone in our town and those nearby were aware that a dance would be held in the Orange Hall on Saturday evening.

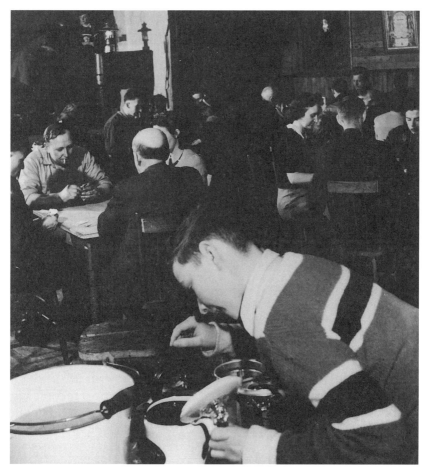

The Orange Hall (1946) is packed with tables of card players enjoying a game of progressive euchre. Red Cross nurse Elsie (Turner) Metcalfe is shown in profile at centre. Jim Miller is seated, facing, in front of the piano. Young Gary Agnew checks out the teapot being kept hot on the box stove, in readiness for refreshment time. *Courtesy Wilberforce Heritage Guild Collection, donated by Red Cross Headquarters, Ottawa.*

That Thursday afternoon another dance committee meeting was being held in our kitchen when the doorbell rang. Aileen answered it and came back all smiles, and loudly announced, "He says he has a sore finger, but I bet he really wants to ask you to go to the dance with him."

When I went out into the hall I recognized Leonard,[3] a tall, dark and handsome bachelor whom I had met at the Marshalls' the previous evening. He had one finger bandaged. "I've had a little accident,"

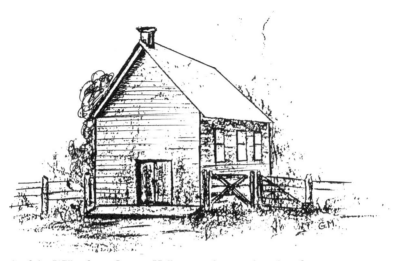

Sketch of the Wilberforce Orange Hall, a popular meeting place for many years. When the Orange Lodge ceased operation for lack of members and interest, Monmouth Township appropriated it for back taxes, had it demolished and replaced with a building to house the Monmouth Library. Original sketch by Gertrude LeRoy Miller.

he said. On examination I found that it had been cut quite badly.

I attended the injury and he was about to leave when he spoke up rather shyly, "Miss LeRoy, may I have the pleasure of your company to the dance Saturday evening?" His charm impressed me. No doubt he had been planning all day on how he could broach the subject. Perhaps that was the cause of his accident. I had no reason to refuse, so as politely as I could (and without laughing), I accepted his invitation. Needless to say, it was a lively dance, enjoyed by everyone. And as the girls had prophesied, I had lots of partners.

As I would be without a car of my own until spring, it was necessary for me to make arrangements for transportation to the different schools. I had been advised that the most logical person to take me would be Tom Marshall. He had a good car and, either he or his stepson Lorne, would always be available. Later, when a car could not be used, anyone requiring my services would have to come for me, or I could hire Sid White, whose wife kept the boarding house. He had horses, a large sleigh, a cutter (a small horse-drawn sleigh) and a democrat (a light wagon), so I should be able to get anywhere under practically any condition. Eventually I tried them all. I would find out about handcars[4] and, in particular, the version called a gas car, later.

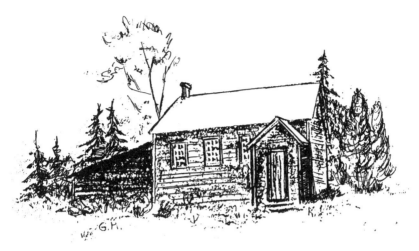

The Cheddar School, known as the "Red School" was a frame building painted red. This was one of the first schools visited by Gertrude LeRoy in the autumn of 1930. Original sketch by Gertrude LeRoy Miller.

It was the understanding that I was to visit all of the twelve schools twice a year if possible. Mr. Marshall advised me that it would be wise to visit the most isolated ones first, and soon, as one never knew when road conditions would prevent access to them until late spring. When we set out for the first one on the list I found out what he meant by "isolated." I still cannot understand why so many of those old schools were built in such remote spots, unless it was that no child should have the advantage of living near the school. The Red School at Cheddar[5] was one these. It was about ten miles from Wilberforce, down the old Burleigh Road over which the pioneers had travelled from Peterborough many years before when seeking a place to settle. The road was also known as the Cheddar Trail. For the first five miles we passed only ten houses. From then on we could see only one through a clearing, but I was told there were quite a few scattered back in the bush. I didn't expect to find many children at school but to my surprise there were twenty-one. What lonely walks those poor children must have had every morning and evening! Some, I learned, had over three miles to come.

The school itself was a desolate-looking building, up on a hill set among rocks and brush, the first rural school I had visited since childhood when my cousin took me to school with her one day while my family was visiting her farm home in southern Ontario. Also, it was the first school of any kind that I had visited alone as a full fledged Public Health Nurse. Needless to say, I was a bit nervous.

Mr. Marshall drove the car as close as possible to the door and stopped, saying, "I'll stay here and catch them as they run out." I asked him to explain what he meant and he told me that the teacher was practically the only stranger that most of the children would have ever seen. They might be frightened at seeing me and run away. I didn't know whether to believe him or not, but by this time the teacher, Mrs. Annie Nesbitt,[6] had heard the car and was at the door. She seemed very glad to see me and, of course knowing the purpose of my visit, asked one of the boys to carry my equipment into the school. This included scales (one of the earliest bathroom models), an awkward homemade gadget for measuring the height of the children. This clever invention consisted of a wooden platform into which I would fit an upright five-foot pole. This pole was marked off in inches and held a sliding piece designed to rest on top of the child's head. (I soon disposed of that complicated and cumbersome piece of equipment and carried a tape measure, which I taped to the door jam with a bit of adhesive tape). As well, there was a suitcase containing records, an eye chart, tongue depressors, toothpicks (for examining the heads) and health literature.

Previous nurses had visited the schools, mainly to try to clean up epidemics of pediculosis (head lice). I've been told that, outside of maternity nursing, one of the greatest blessings brought about by the Red Cross Nursing Services was the riddance of head and body lice from the schools. The majority of the men were in logging camps during the winters and living in very close proximity with others, many of whom were transients. It was only natural that one person with head or body lice was all that was necessary to spread the pestilence throughout the camp. As the men had no way of getting rid of them until they were home to stay, it didn't take long for the condition to spread throughout the household, then the school. I ran across a few cases, but my predecessors had them pretty well cleaned up, though a few families had to be checked frequently.

The children didn't take this problem as seriously as the parents. One adult told me that when he was a schoolboy, head lice was so common with some families that the other children made a real joke of the problem. The boys would pick them off the girls in front of them and race them across a sheet of paper. They would kill the slow ones and put the winners back, to improve the breed!

Well, here I was at my first school. The teacher introduced me to the children and I spoke to them for a minute or so, explaining the purpose of my visit and procedure. Advising them to carry on with their regular work, I indicated that each would be called, one at a time. I set up my equipment at the back of the room, placed the eye chart on one wall, measured 20 feet back and marked where the child would stand for an eye test.

Besides checking vision, hearing, weight and height, the routine included inspection of the skin on hands, arms and neck for any signs of a rash or sores. Throats, mouths, and teeth were checked for any suggestion of diseased tonsils, sores, decay or any other abnormalities. Hair and scalp were examined for head lice or sores. Posture was noted. All findings were recorded on individual cards, which I kept on file. Any defect found would also be written on a special form and sent home to the parents. Later, when I had a car of my own and time permitted, I would deliver these personally and discuss the matter of treatment with the parents.

When I had finished the inspections, I gave the children a little health talk, followed by the reading of a little story containing a health lesson. They weren't a bit frightened and seemed to enjoy my visit.

While planning for my next trip, I noticed by my map that there were two schools about four miles apart, so I decided to do both in one day. It would mean being away from the Outpost for that time, but I decided to take the chance. Mr. Marshall dropped me off at the first school before nine o'clock and said he would visit some friends in the nearby town, make arrangements for our lunch and call for me at noon. With thirty-six pupils at this school, I had plenty to keep me busy until noon. I was ready for a meal when Mr. Marshall retrieved me.

Since coming to this vicinity, I had learned that most families raised and butchered their own pigs, and that pork was about the only meat they ate. Occasionally, they would have beef or kill a deer, but pork and potatoes constituted their staple diet. In order to keep the pork during the summer, they salted it or kept it in brine. To prepare it for eating, the pork had to be par-boiled to remove the salt. Well, our hostess for that day evidently forgot to prepare the pork she fried for us. Perhaps she became excited when she learned that the new nurse was coming for dinner. It was also so fat, as well as salty, we could hardly swallow it. Possibly they liked pork that way, but we didn't. Along with the salt pork, we had plain boiled potatoes and gravy made by adding only water to the fat drippings from the meat. However, there were lots of homemade bread and butter, raisin pie, cookies and tea. All-in-all we really did very well.

With only twenty-seven children at the next school, the health inspection didn't take quite so long and we were back at the Outpost shortly after 4 p.m. Despite the quite strenuous day I had enjoyed it and felt that I was really making some headway with my work. Later, another school on my list, Hotspur,[7] in a very isolated area, had only three pupils, so that site did not take much of my time. Shortly after my next visit there, it was closed and the children were taken in to school at Tory Hill.

During my course in Public Health Nursing, I'd had a month of fieldwork in an eastern Ontario town where school nursing was a major part of the program. I had also visited Toronto schools during my senior year in training, so these routine school visits were not likely to present any new problems, so I thought. Well, my first year or so in this part of the country certainly provided what is now called "on the job" education. Some of these "learning opportunities," such as dealing with individual cups brought from home, roller towels and hand washing procedures, helped strengthen my coping skills.

In the school Health Program, although the children were supposed to be my main concern, I frequently wondered about the teachers, particularly those who were teaching in the most isolated places. Most were young women, some mere girls teaching for the first time. Some may never have been away from home before. What kind of homes were they boarding in? I suspected that the conditions in some of these homes were anything but pleasant. Their boarding places were usually arranged by local school boards, with either the secretary or chairman winning the draw and thus the benefit of the teacher's board money. And there they would be stuck, perhaps seeing no other family from one week to the next.

One teacher told me about her boarding place, at the home of the board secretary, a man with a large family. It was a fairly big house and she had a small room to herself upstairs. A stovepipe ran up through from the bedroom downstairs which the parents occupied. One night she was awakened by considerable commotion. Hearing the cries of a new baby, she realized the cause and was horrified when she found out that there was no doctor, no nurse, or even a neighbour. The husband had looked after everything as (she learned later) he had always done at such times!

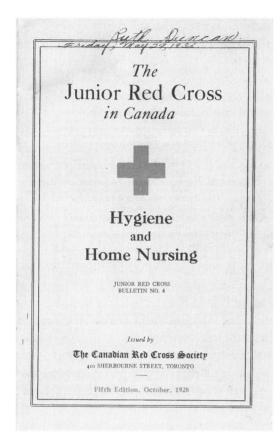

Cover of "The Junior Red Cross" manual, 1928. The text outlines lessons for boys and girls together but specifies for Sections 5 and 6 that the girls will take "Home Nursing" and "Care of the Baby," while the boys take "Camp Sanitation" and "Camp Cooking." Red Cross buttons (pins) were given out to the students each year. *Courtesy Wilberforce Heritage Guild Collection.*

How fortunate I was to be in a village, even if it was small, and free to move about my large territory rather than being confined to a small school section in the backwoods. I wondered what I might do to make the social lives of these girls a little brighter. Most schools I would not be visiting again until late spring when the roads dried up sufficiently for a car to travel safely. Actually, my first opportunity to do something, I realized, was close at hand. Was I not on the committee to help plan the Halloween Masquerade Dance? Why not invite the teachers from out-of-town to spend the weekend with us? What better way of getting acquainted with each other than by living together for a couple of days? Aileen was agreeable so I sent out the invitations and crossed my fingers, hoping that we would admit no patients in the meantime. If that were the case, however, the neighbours offered to help out.

The teachers were to arrive in time for the Friday dance, after which they would sleep at the Outpost. Our sleeping accommodation consisted of four hospital beds and one single cot, but who cared? We would be very late getting to bed anyway and, after all, most of the girls would have nothing to do for the next seven weekends but sleep. Hence, two or three to a bed wasn't even a concern. The dance was a huge success and everyone had a happy fun-filled evening.

On Saturday afternoon we all gathered in the Outpost living room where we held a real Teacher-Nurse Conference and discussed matters that concerned both us and the children we were serving. I told them all I knew about Junior Red Cross[8] and gave them some literature I had secured for the occasion. For me, and I am sure for the teachers as well, the discussions were very inspiring and helpful.

After lunch some went for walks while others caught up on their sleep, then we all played cards until supper time. The young men of the town had decided that having all those extra girls in town was too good an opportunity to miss, so they organized another dance for Saturday night. So the teachers not only enjoyed a pleasant weekend, but also were provided with delightful memories to recall during the dull winter evenings ahead. Incidentally, Junior Red Cross was started in several schools following our little conference.

Another memorable weekend was soon to follow, but it did not leave such happy memories. It was a beautiful Sunday afternoon. The Marshalls decided to go for a drive, invited me to accompany them and asked if there were any calls I would like to make. As it happened, there was one in particular. I had visited Kennaway School recently and found a child about whom I was quite concerned. When I indicated that I would welcome an opportunity to talk to her parents, we struck out in that direction.

One interesting stretch of road we covered was known as the Long Crossway, a corduroy road. It had been built by laying logs transversely side by side for over half a mile through a swamp. There was a slight curve about half way along, but even so it was the longest stretch of straight road I'd seen so far in this country.

When we finally reached our destination, the sight that met us was appalling! There was nothing but smoldering ruins of the home![9] Some men from the neighbourhood were poking around among the hot ashes and they told us what they knew. As this was a very sparsely settled area, there were no near neighbours, so by the time the fire had been seen it was too late to save anything. All the occupants were severely burned and had been taken to Bancroft Red Cross Hospital (much larger and better equipped than the one at Wilberforce). The most critically burned, they said, were two little girls (both died later). It was thought that the fire had been caused by a coal oil lamp, which had been left burning at night and had possibly been turned up too high. This was my first taste of tragedy.

4

Books Bring Prince Charming and Other Charming Customs

One Saturday Aileen had gone out for the evening and I was alone reading when the doorbell rang. There stood a tall dark man about my age, a complete stranger to me. "Miss LeRoy?"

"Yes."

"I'm Delbert Miller. I'm wondering if you have any interesting books in the library that I could read. I'm home from the camp for the weekend with nothing to do." (Didn't Aileen say he would find an excuse?)

"The books all look very old to me," I replied. "But you might be able to find something interesting. Come in and look them over."

He did, and eventually found a couple he thought he might like. After explaining the proper spelling of his name as I wrote it down (A'Delbert) I decided he was really more interested in getting aquainted with the nurse than in finding something to read. I didn't mind, for we spcnt a very pleasant evening discussing the beauty and natural resources of the area. To me, he seemed to be a real outdoors man. Del said he had a canoe and would like to take me up to Grace Lake the next afternoon where I would see some really beautiful scenery.

Well, I never again had to wonder about a partner for a dance. Incidentally, he did the calling[1] for many of them. From then on he came

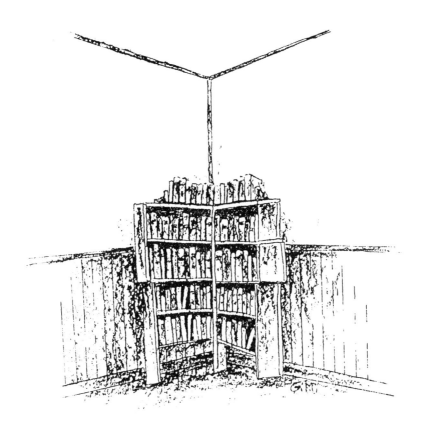

Some books on shelves in one corner of the Outpost living room. It is likely they were collected by Volunteer Red Cross Groups in Toronto and donated to this rural community. No doubt this gift of books was much appreciated. Original sketch by Gertrude LeRoy Miller.

home every weekend and the canoe found a permanent parking place on our beach. I now had one more reason for liking this place.

I was interested in learning from Del how several of the lakes had been stocked with fish. Both he and his father worked in sawmills during the summers, as his father was a sawyer. Del worked as a setter, that is, he rode on the carriage that carried the log up to the saw and kept working the levers which turned the log and regulated the thickness of each board, in response to signals from the sawyer. During the evenings the men would set out nets in the lake around the mill and catch small fish. Saturday night they would bring them home in milk cans, on the "pede," and with the help of friends, would carry them

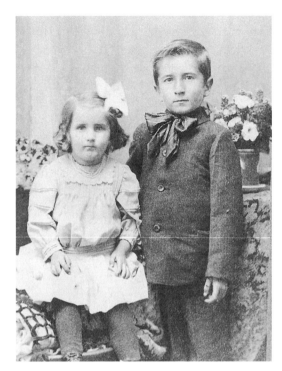

A young A'Delbert Miller (about six years of age) formally photographed with his sister Mary. Delbert later married the Red Cross Outpost Hospital nurse, Gertrude. Mary would marry and become Mrs. Alfred Dunford. *Courtesy Wilberforce Heritage Guild Collection.*

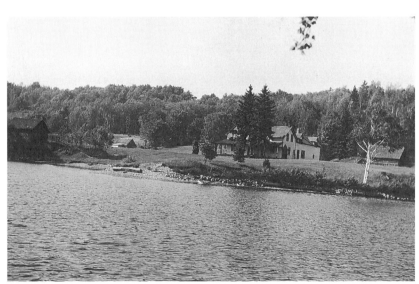

This postcard scene is of Dark Lake (formerly Pusey Lake) on which the Outpost backed. Delbert would have paddled his canoe through this waterway to take Gertrude to Grace Lake. The house shown was the home of John Holmes, located just northeast of the Outpost. *Courtesy Agnew Family Collection.*

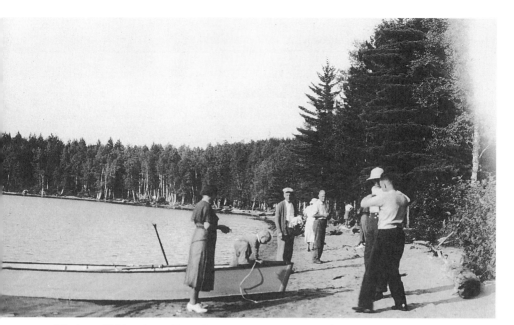

The beautiful beach on Grace Lake was the destination, for many years, for picnics planned by families such as shown in this group. Just a paddle up the Grace River, and through the channel was one of the prettiest lakes in Ontario. *Courtesy Agnew Family Collection.*

to various lakes. The pede was a three-wheeled velocipede,[2] which was propelled along the railroad tracks by means of hand pumping. They owned the vehicle and had permission to use it on the tracks, as there was no other way of getting home except to walk. In those days men worked six full days a week.

We spent many pleasant Sunday afternoons paddling around Dark Lake and up the picturesque [Grace] river to beautiful Grace Lake, with its broad sand beach, the favourite picnic spot of the community. Sometimes we would do a bit of fishing, a new sport for me. What I most enjoyed was the peaceful silence. Del was an expert canoeist and could paddle without making a sound to disturb any wildlife around the water's edge or among the tall reeds. Often we would see fish jumping out of the water to catch a fly, a deer drinking, or a mink running over the rocks and into the water. Once we came across a family of otter at play, most interesting entertainment indeed.

Just "listening" to the silence was tranquilizing medicine. Here we were, about 1400 feet above sea level and surrounded by colourful hills. A loon, calling to its mate, would light on the water not far away.

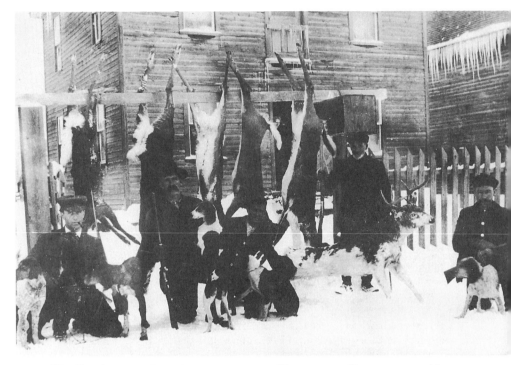

The "hunting season" was important to many. Here a party of hunters pose with their "catch" in the early 1900s. Hunting was more than just sport. Venison would be the principal source of meat for many households for some time. George Miller's house is in the background. *Courtesy Wilberforce Heritage Guild Collection.*

As we watched, it would dive completely underneath and for several minutes there would be no sign of the bird. At last it would appear a great distance away. I had never seen a loon before. Del told me what odd birds they are, with legs so short they cannot rise into the air from land. Their nests are usually on bare ground or rocks close to the water. He told me of an experience he had as a boy. He found a loon's nest and, just for fun, took one of the eggs home and slipped it into a whole nest under one of his mother's brooding hens. One day the whole barnyard was in an uproar! The loon had hatched and was making so much noise it had frightened all the hens! My education was certainly expanding in many ways since I had come closer to nature.

Earlier that first fall I learned that just as the I.B.&O. supposedly ran on a calendar schedule rather than by the clock, this community referred to "Hunting Season" rather than the standard seasonal calendar. This was a focal point of the year. Such and such an incident happened so many weeks before or after hunting season. In spite of the fact that this particular season lasted for only two weeks in early November, it seemed to be the main topic of conversation whenever two or more men got together from about October first until after Christmas. They would have the details and highlights of the last hunt to go over as well as many others of past years. Perhaps someone had seen deer tracks in an unusual place, so a new "runway" was discovered. Rifles would be getting an extra polishing and target practice would be the chief pastime. Hounds would be bought, sold, or traded and there would be a general air of excitement working up as the days of actual hunting drew near.

All of this excitement and activity did not concern the men alone, for no matter which home one visited, the housewives seemed to be up to their ears in baking for the hunters. There would be cookies by the hundreds, fruitcakes, and pies of every description, preserves, pickles, loaves of bread and crocks of butter. I decided that the men must eat a great deal more food while hunting than at any other time, but I guess it involved very strenuous work. Many friends came from the cities to hunt with them.

Along in November Aileen introduced me to the mail order catalogues.[3] What a wonderful way to do one's Christmas shopping! Other years I would battle my way through crowds on street cars and then more crowds in stores, and look by the hour, only to return home almost empty-handed, and have to go through it all again. This was so simple and intriguing. We could just sit in a nice warm room, turn the magic pages and pick out just what we wanted. We could change our minds a dozen times before actually sending for the articles and, if we were not satisfied with the goods when they arrived, they could easily be exchanged. Just think of all the car fare saved. So every spare moment for weeks before Christmas was spent studying catalogues.

About this time it was customary for the teachers and children to start planning for their Christmas concerts. Every school must have one and every child must take part, either in song, recitation, play or chorus. Every spare moment for weeks would be spent practising. There were costumes to sew and posters to make and send out to all surrounding villages where they would be displayed in post offices and stores. Great care would be taken to ensure that no two concerts were held the same evening because everybody tried to attend as many as possible. A lively dance usually followed each concert, after, of course, a visit from Santa who distributed presents, with candy and an orange for each child, including each baby. The chairs would then be pushed back against the walls and a fiddler would start tuning up and in no time one would hear, "Come on now, four more couples,–four more couples here,–two more couples here,"…and away they'd go! One just about had to keep on dancing because most of the chairs would be laden down with sleeping children or piled high with winter wraps. Just when you are about ready to drop, on comes the food. Cups would be passed around and then the men would appear with huge jugs of steaming hot tea, followed by sandwiches, cake and cookies of every description. It would be in the wee small hours when one arrived home, but it was the holiday season and there were still a few hours to rest before leaving for the next concert. For the Nurse, however, business came before pleasure. That first Christmas I managed to take in only one and a half concerts.

I had accepted Del's invitation to accompany him to the Tory Hill concert, seven miles away. As there was lots of snow, he arranged to borrow a horse and cutter from Walter Clark down the road. I was thrilled indeed, not so much with the prospects of the concert and dance, as with the cutter ride. I had not had a ride in a cutter since I was a child visiting my grandparents. Well did I remember the buffalo robe and the jingling sleigh bells on the trotting horse, as we slid along so smoothly over the snow-covered roads.

Del was to call for me about seven o'clock, but at 5:30 the I.B.&O. brought us a visitor! She had come from Gooderham and was a stranger to me. She informed me that her baby was due to arrive that night. It was her first baby and so far she'd had no pains and was feeling fine but thought she would be safer at the Outpost. I admitted her and when I mentioned "doctor" she said, "Oh, no. I don't think a doctor will be necessary now that I'm here."

I did all the routine examining and questioning and decided her condition seemed to be normal. But I didn't know what to do about leaving her in Aileen's care for the evening. I figured that, this being her first baby, if labour had not begun by seven o'clock she would be safe to leave until near midnight. I decided to slip over and see what Mrs. Marshall thought of the situation. She was the mother of nine and was always ready with a helping hand or a bit of advice. She told me to go by all means. She knew the patient and would go over during the evening and visit her. If she should need me she would send word, so away we went. I need not have worried as the patient was sound asleep when I returned, and her baby not born until late the next night.

Well, the concert and the cutter ride with the sleigh bells jingling surpassed all my expectations. And we did not upset in a snowbank on our way home, as Del's young brother Jimmy, reported to his school chums the next day. He was just trying to get even with Del for teasing him about Santa Claus.

Some time before this Jimmy had come home from school and told his folks, "You're not going to fool me anymore! There isn't any Santa Claus! The kids all said so! So you don't need to think you can fool me anymore."

As Christmas drew near, Del said to him one day, "Well, Jimmy, I guess you've been too smart this year. You say there is no Santa Claus, so I guess you won't be getting any presents. Too bad, because you sure got a lot last year."

Poor fellow was worried sick. This time he'd put his foot in it! Why hadn't he kept quiet? His Christmas would be spoiled for sure. However, there must be some way he could work it out yet, so when he got his mother alone he told her he didn't believe a word of what the kids had told him about Santa Claus. He then decided to get even with his brother for teasing him. When he went to school the morning after the Tory Hill concert he told the boys that his brother Delbert thought he was pretty smart when he got the nurse to go to the concert with him, but he wasn't so smart when the cutter upset in a snowbank.

When the night arrived for the Wilberforce school concert, being held in the Orange Hall just across the road, Aileen and I took turns going back and forth. Both of us were delighted to have a mother and baby to care for at Christmas. When we learned that the patient didn't have many comforts at home, we took great pleasure in playing Santa to her, as did our neighbours.

Our town that Christmas morning looked just like a picture on a Christmas card. A fresh blanket of pure white snow covered everything. The snow covered boughs of the evergreens were bent low and each fence post had a new six-inch cap. The road was a perfectly smooth white blanket except for a sleigh track down the centre. Santa's, no doubt! Across the way the hill looked perfect for tobogganing or skiing, and before long it was being put to good use as youngsters began trying out their new equipment.

One afternoon during the Christmas holidays we had a party for the small children of the community. Some friends in the city had very kindly sent a large box of toys and clothing for me to share among

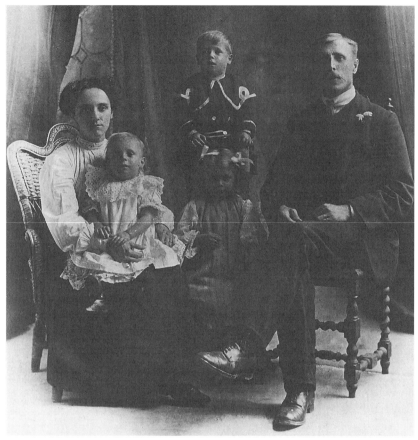

A formal family portrait of Clara and Frank Schofield taken in England. Reg sits on his mother's knee, Frank Jr is behind his sister Doris, circa 1910. *Courtesy Wilberforce Heritage Guild Collection, donated by the Schofield family.*

the children. After I bought candy, nuts and fruit, Aileen and I made and filled Christmas stockings to go around. The children played games, had lunch, then Santa (Frank Schofield) arrived, huffing and puffing in his red suit, and distributed the gifts. Judging by the noise they made, a good time was had by all!

Mr. Schofield, I might say, was the real pillar of the Red Cross in Wilberforce. He was a war veteran and was the Treasurer/Secretary of the Red Cross Committee for many years. It was his brother, Alfred, whose efforts brought the Outpost Hospital into being in the first place. Frank and his boys, Frank and Reg, were always on hand when a job of any kind was to be done. His only daughter[4] who had worked as a housekeeper for a previous nurse, had gone on to high school in

Haliburton and was now about to graduate and become a Registered Nurse in Lindsay.

Activities in the town changed as winter progressed. Once the Christmas holidays were over everything seemed to quieten down, with most of the men gone off to logging camps and the children back at school. It was then that the mothers would get at their knitting in real earnest. And how those needles did fly! Plenty of warm woollen socks and mitts for the men were most important, for it was mighty cold working in far below zero weather. And the children, too, needed their cosy socks, mitts and sweaters.

When the snow was getting deeper and deeper, and the mercury beginning to drop almost out of sight, I found that something had to be done about hiking clothes. Most of my calls had to be made on foot. A fur coat and overshoes were fine for riding in a vehicle or even walking along cleared paths, but not even the roads were plowed those days. I had noticed that the older girls wore heavy riding breeches so I invested in a pair, along with a leather jacket and heavy boots large enough for extra wool socks. Once I oiled the boots to make them waterproof, I was all set to go calling. I may not have been a perfect model in that outfit, but it enabled me to get on with my work.

For those icy trips on the gas car [handcar] or by sleigh, I had an entirely different outfit. After rummaging about in an old trunk in the storeroom I had found a big fur cap which I could pull down over my forehead and ears and a pair of very large fur lined boots made for warmth, not walking. These I could pull on over my overshoes. With my own fur coat and a heavy woollen blanket to wrap around my legs, I never suffered from the cold on any of my long trips.

For variety, after most of their knitting was finished, the women would get out their quilt patches and try to make at least one quilt before spring. Some were really beautiful while others were made purely for warmth. One grandmother showed me quilts she had made for each of her children and her grandchildren, nineteen in all. All her quilts were beautiful. Later there would be a round of quilting bees, all day events for the women, when it was hard to tell what went faster, the tongues or the needles. One must remember, there were no telephones and so much to talk about!

I was fortunate in owning one of the only two radios in town that first winter. We used it very sparingly as it ran on a car battery, which had to be sent by train to Bancroft to be re-charged. We listened to the news, *Amos 'n Andy*, and, of course, the hockey games every Satur-

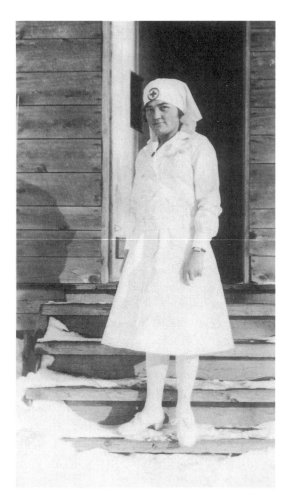

Gertrude LeRoy in uniform during her first winter (1930–31) as the Red Cross Outpost nurse, standing on the steps of the Wilberforce Outpost Hospital. *Courtesy Wilberforce Heritage Guild Collection.*

day night. For the latter we always had a fair-sized audience, and it was every bit as exciting, I'm sure, as it was right at the game. Everyone would be sitting on the edge of the chair, constantly creeping closer and closer until at the end of a period we would be crowded around the radio. Some of us women were knitting stockings for a local family and the more exciting the game, the faster we would knit. I'm sure the squeals and yells as Foster Hewitt shouted, "He shoots! He scores!" could be heard almost to Tory Hill! There was still an audience the night Ken Doherty scored the winning goal at 2 a.m.

If the weather permitted, often the boys would clear off a rink on the lake for skating and, in spite of many handicaps, played many exciting games of hockey. Even young Ernie Tallman became famous

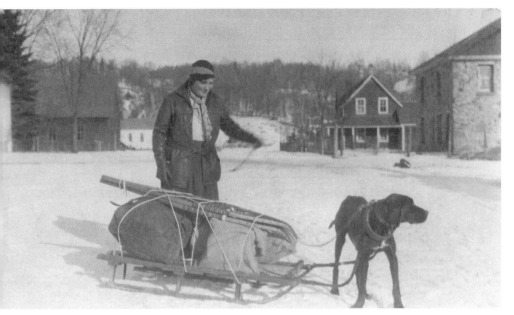

No matter the season or weather, the Red Cross nurse had to be prepared to venture out to her patients. Though this sleigh was known to be packed by Del Miller in preparation for a trapping trip, Gertrude did, at times, travel by dog sleigh. This dog, named Jack, belonged to the Walter Clark family. Note Gertrude's clothing and the snowshoes. *Courtesy Wilberforce Heritage Guild Collection, donated by Aileen Ames Walker.*

as a juvenile Foster Hewitt. He would use his time off to "broadcast" to the world around him, the activities of the players and one could often hear him shout, "He shoots! He scores!"

When I found out how much the people enjoyed playing euchre, we arranged to have card parties at the Outpost every couple of weeks, except when we had a patient. We charged twenty-five cents each and used the proceeds to purchase articles needed at the Outpost. These parties went over in a big way. Sometimes we had as many as ten tables, with people coming from other communities.

One of the things I noticed during my first winter spent in Wilber-force, was the lack of reading material. Few newspapers circulated except the *Family Herald* and the weekly local *Minden Echo*. I subscribed to a Toronto daily paper which, because of the train service, came only three times a week. Of course, in those days a paper a few days old was still news and was passed along. I had heard about the Travelling Library Service, so introduced it to our village. This proved a great boon to the community, especially to the young people who were the most interested in reading, but it provided a variety of good reading for everyone on a monthly basis.

Tobogganing was the rage when there was lots of snow and all ages took part. The hill behind the school was an ideal spot for the sport, but gradually this gave way to skiing. Some Finlanders cutting cordwood a few miles away had made their own skis to travel back and forth. The locals greatly admired their skill in handling them and soon most of the young people and children had their own. It certainly was the way to get around when the snow was too deep for walking. I tried skiis a few times but decided they were too fast for me, so I turned to snowshoes, which I soon learned to handle quite well.

During the first winter in this community I learned many things first hand, causing me to wonder if those who wrote textbooks or taught health courses had gained their knowledge merely by hearsay. For instance, the children were supposed to be taught that they should always sleep with their windows open, both winter and summer. Well, that might be sensible if they lived in steam heated apartments in the city, but I learned from my own experience that first winter, how impractical that idea was.

At the Outpost we were reasonably comfortable during the day when we were there to keep feeding the stove and furnace, and if the wind was not blowing too hard. We did not notice the draughts around the windows and doors, much. But at night when the fires were low or out, well, we needed no open windows to provide fresh air!

Our furnace, incidentally, had been built to burn coal. A few years previously someone on the "Committee" had a chance to buy it at a reasonable price, so here it was. It was a priceless affair so all the heat it provided was channelled through a large square grate directly above it, which happened to be in the hall between the living room and the front doors. So, on very cold days we could always absorb some of the heat by standing on the grate. Having been designed for coal, the furnace door was merely large enough to accommodate a scoop shovel. And the firebox itself, instead of being suited to large chunks of cord wood, was round and deep. Therefore, the wood had to be cut short and split into small pieces so it could be packed tightly together on end. That way it burned much faster so had to be stoked more often. I soon found out what an intricate task it was to put wood in and stand it up without touching the hot door! City life had certainly not trained me for these early morning jaunts to the dark cellar. Frequently we would take turns going down during the night. Often on extremely cold mornings the very welcome sound of a man's footsteps could be heard descending this cavern and then of the furnace being stoked. We never locked our doors and one of our neighbours, after looking after his own heat, would slip over and get our place warmed up.

Yes, we were well looked after, and at least we could keep warm. But how must those people who were living in old log houses or rough buildings where there were plenty of visible cracks stand it! At forty to fifty degrees below zero fahrenheit, with strong winds rattling our windows, it was tough for us. But how were they managing, especially the children! I had seen many houses where quilts or cardboard were covering windows in place of glass to keep out the cold, and I'm sure there were some who hadn't enough quilts to keep them warm in bed.

Needless to say, I never again included "Sleeping with the windows open" among the rules of health, especially when referring to winter. However, lessons on cleanliness were certainly needed in most of the schools, as there were usually a few families who seemingly made little effort to be clean. According to the health rules, everyone should have at least one full bath each week. I did my best to teach the importance of personal cleanliness. But when I realized what a problem it must be for a large family living in two or three rooms to find enough privacy to have even a sponge bath after having to carry water, possibly a quarter of a mile, well, no wonder they or their clothing were not always clean.

5

Getting There in Winter
is Half the Task

The roads throughout Monmouth Township in this day and age[1] are well travelled during both winter and summer, regardless of the depth of snow on the land. Results of blizzards or snowstorms are cleared as quickly as up-to-date equipment can arrive on the scene. The situation was very different in the early 1930s when many of the roads were mere widened cow paths winding around rocks and lakes, over hills and through the woods, and never plowed during the winter. Once the snow came, shortcuts were taken over frozen lakes and fields.

Wilberforce was completely isolated from the outside world during the winters, except for the I.B.&O. train service three times a week. The tracks were always kept clear and provided good walking conditions in two directions.

Regardless of road conditions people did get sick and babies were born, and the purpose of my being there was to help. My first real taste of winter transportation was one to be remembered. It was late January and very cold and windy, and it had been snowing all day. I went to bed as usual, hoping there would be no calls until the storm was over. About one o'clock I woke up with a start, thinking I could hear sleigh bells over the noise of the wind and sleet striking the win-

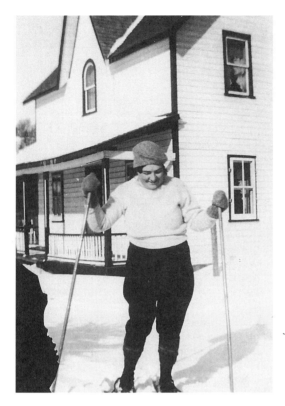

Gertrude LeRoy tries out skis. The home of William and Isabel Shay in the background, is the house immediately north of the Wilberforce Outpost. The photograph may have been taken by Mr. Shay, an uncle of Aileen Ames. *Courtesy Wilberforce Heritage Guild Collection, donated by Aileen Ames Walker.*

dow. I lit my lamp and was wondering whether I should get dressed, when a noise was heard at the front door, like someone stamping the snow off his feet, then came the doorbell. A man covered with snow and ice, who introduced himself as Bill B., said his wife was having a baby. Would I please come with him? I assured him I would be ready in a jiffy and invited him in to get warm while I dressed.

We were soon on our way in his cutter, wrapped in blankets to our chins. What a night! Snow, sleet and wind! His former tracks were almost completely obliterated and we could barely see the road. And the poor horse did not seem a bit anxious to make the trip. Every few minutes she would stop and it would require a great deal of coaxing to get her to go on. We were very desirous of making good time as Bill said his wife was alone except for their seven-year-old daughter. He explained that the horse belonged to a friend in Essonville, in the opposite direction, and that he was keeping her for the winter in order to have her for this particular occasion. Coming to the Outpost, she thought she was on her way home so wasted no time. Now that the

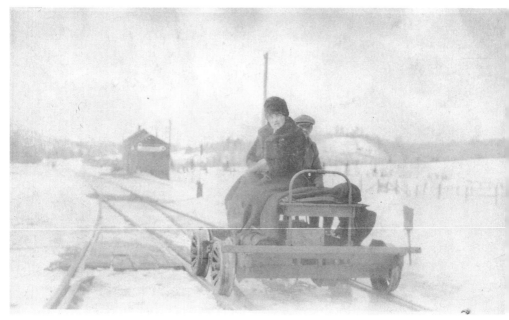

Dressed in a fur coat, over lots of other clothes, Gertrude LeRoy is prepared for a cold ride on the jigger (handcar), on her way to visit a patient. Note the Wilber-force Station in the background and the open fields. The setting is near the intersection of the I.B.&O. Railway and the Burleigh Road. *Courtesy Wilberforce Heritage Guild Collection, donated by Reg and Winnie Schofield and family.*

mare was going back she decided to balk! And in a race with the stork!

Incidentally, this was the same road I had travelled to my first case in the old Model T. The hills were still there, as steep as ever, only now they were drifted with snow and we were almost blinded by the sleet and wind. I prayed just as hard, not so much for a safe trip, but that I might reach the patient in time to help her. Finally, when the horse absolutely refused to go another step despite the urging, Bill got out and led for at least a mile. At last we reached the home of my very first patient, but still some distance to go. Bill led the mare to the stable and showed me the way to go in and get warm. He went on into the house to rouse the owner and arranged to borrow one of his horses to take us the remaining two or so miles.

I was surprised to find the stable so warm and cozy. With several cows and three horses in this old building, and with snow banked up around the outside and tons of hay in the loft overhead, it would be almost as warm as the house with its two stoves.

In a short time we were on our way, and with much better speed.

While the patient was certainly glad to see us, the baby didn't arrive until about three hours later. When finally I had the mother fixed up, bed made, and baby bathed and tucked in his basket, the sun was shining. I looked out the window and could see nothing but snowdrifts. How would I get home? Bill had been out to do his chores and said it was very cold, but the wind had died down. Their daughter, Sally, would not try to go to school as it was too far to walk through the snow, but he thought we could make it through to Wilberforce with horse and cutter. Not liking the idea of leaving the mother and baby with just a seven-year-old child for so long, I decided not to be in a hurry about starting out. We were at the table eating our oatmeal porridge when I glanced out the window and saw a team and sleigh turning up the lane.

"Company's coming," I shouted.

"Sure enough," Bill said, as he jumped up to look. "Why, that's Wilfred Croft coming for Mr. Webber's hay, I bet you!" Grabbing his coat and cap, he hurried out to meet him. I called to him, suggesting that I wouldn't mind riding on top of the load if he'd let me. I knew he would be going right past the Outpost. Someone was looking after me for sure.

The men didn't think I would like that, but I told them I thought it would be fun. When they finished loading, they put up a ladder and up I climbed. Once settled in a nice warm nest on top of the load, I was as comfortable "as a bug in a rug."

What a ride it was, up and down hill. Several times I thought we would upset! Frequently I had to dodge tree branches. And going down the steep hills, I was afraid we would slide into the horses. Amazingly, we reached town safe and sound, but I was very disappointed that not one person was around to see me as we drove down the main street! The next question was how was I to get down? We had gone right on to the Webber barn at the end of town. The simplest way, I decided, was to slide off into a snowbank, so that is what I did.

One other very cold evening a few weeks later, I was introduced to another means of transportation, one I was to depend on many times. Some friends had dropped in and we were having a game of dominoes. Every few minutes there was a loud "bang," and we knew the frost had loosened another clapboard on the building. How nice it was to be able to stay in and keep warm! I had not been called out for several days. Everyone was quite healthy it seemed.

About eleven o'clock that night we heard footsteps on the front

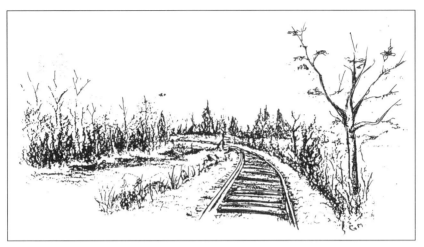

The Irondale, Bancroft and Ottawa rail line. Original sketch by Gertrude LeRoy Miller.

porch, then the doorbell. It was Mr. Agnew with a message for me, to please go to Gooderham as soon as possible by gas car. I would be met at the station and taken to the patient, who was having a baby. Of course I had never heard of the people before, but that meant nothing. Also, I had never had a ride on the gas car[2] before either, but it was the only possible mode of transportation at this time, as the roads were blocked with snow. The tracks were always kept clear.

There was quite a mad scramble for a few minutes. Del rushed down to the Station House to make arrangements with Ben Wright, the Section Foreman, and to help get the car on the track and running. In the meantime I put on all the warm clothing I could find, for it was 28 degrees (F) below zero. In a short time there was quite a parade trudging single file through the snow from the Outpost down to the railway track. I was so padded with clothing that I was thankful not to have to carry anything. Someone had the big suitcase, another the black bag, one had the big blanket, and yet another the big fur boots.

When we reached the tracks, the men had the car out and were trying to start the engine. The gas car was the vehicle which the section men used to patrol the tracks, and was merely a platform on wheels with a large tool box down the centre and gasoline engine at one end. An iron bar extended over the top from one end to the other. I was instructed to sit on the box with my back against the bar (I also hung onto it to keep from sliding off), and rest my feet on the six or so inches of platform below. I put my feet into the fur boots, wrapped

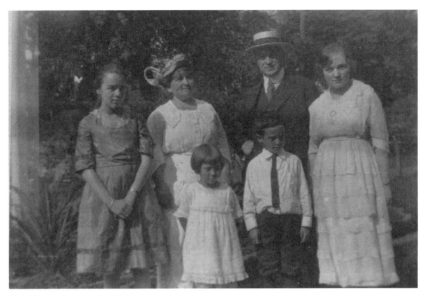

Charles and Emma (McCoubrey) LeRoy and family shown in 1919. Reta is to the left beside her mother; Virginia and Donald are in front; Gertrude is to the right beside her father. *Courtesy Virginia (LeRoy) Luckock.*

the blanket snugly around me, took the black bag on my lap and settled down for I didn't know what.

They finally got the engine started and we were off. Del, with his father's big fur-lined coat which he had picked up on the way, sat in front of me and held a lantern. Ben stood at the back and operated the engine. What a ride! I shall never forget it, though I have ridden on the gas car dozens of times since, both night and day. The lantern didn't light up much of the countryside or even the track, as we sped along at I don't know what speed, but seemed to me like a bullet being shot through the darkness. The men didn't seem to be worrying, so I tried to put aside my fears and think of the patient who was waiting for me. Twice we had to stop and fill the radiator with snow, and finally with water at a spring, all because, in the excitement, the men forgot to fill the rad before we left. We sped on through cuts with high walls of rock on either side, then over bridges where there seemed to be nothing but the rails between us and deep gorges below.

Finally, we saw a light and hoped it would be the station at Gooderham. As we slowed and stopped, I could see a team of horses hitched to a bobsleigh heaped with straw. A wide board arrangement was across the centre and a pile of quilts. I was instructed to sit between quilts and rest my back against the board. Once more we were off. Two men accompanied the team and sleigh, and I learned that one was the patient's husband. He informed me that his mother and a neighbour were with his wife but no doctor had been called. They were all sure, he said, that no doctor would be neeeded when they were able to get me! That did inspire me to send up another little prayer for wisdom and help from the Great Physician. So far he had never failed me.

We jogged along for half an hour or so, a far more comfortable ride than on the gas car, then turned off the road into a short lane toward a house that was well lit up. I awkwardly crawled out of my soft bed and jumped off the sleigh into the snow. By then the door was open and an elderly woman escorted me into the kitchen where I removed all of my heavy togs; then into the front room and the patient.

After examining her, I realized that about another half-hour and the stork would have won the race. However, I could tell that these women had experienced similar situations before, as little was left for me to do regarding preparations. Before long, a bouncing baby girl arrived safely and everyone was happy.

The patient's husband, after an early breakfast, drove me to the station and the Gooderham section man took me back to Wilberforce on his gas car. The return ride in broad daylight was thrilling, but nothing like it had been before, speeding through the dark of the night.

My parents[3] had visited me twice since my arrival at Wilberforce and were quite satisfied that I was safe and sound and happy in doing work that I enjoyed. And they too fell in love with the country. My sister, Reta, decided she would like to come from Toronto and see for herself, so planned to come and spend Easter with me. Everything had been quiet around the Outpost for a week or two and not being aware of anything coming up, I decided to take part of a day off and go meet her.

Now, our railway system requires considerable explanation. In the first place, as I've mentioned before, the train only ran three days a week: Monday, Wednesday, and Friday. Its starting point was Bancroft, about 25 miles to the northeast, as the crow flies. It left there, or was supposed to, around 8:30 a.m. but by the time it had stopped at various sidings and stations to pick up cars, take water, load freight…, it was usually eleven o'clock or later when it puffed into our station. After a half-hour there, backing up, going foreward, puffing, tooting, the train would pant up a long grade and finally pick up its top speed of fifteen miles per hour, and so on to the next station. At Gooderham, it stopped for an hour while the trainmen and any passengers who wished, went into the station house dining room for a hot meal. I had eaten lunch before leaving so had an hour to relax. A few miles further on we came to Howland Junction, which, as I have explained earlier, is where we meet the train from Lindsay and switch engines.

The Lindsay train was waiting for us. It meant that I would have to leave this coach, go over to the other track and board the other one on which Reta had travelled and which we would take back to Wilberforce. However, just as I stepped off, a man spoke to me, asking if I was the nurse from Wilberforce. I assured him that I was, wondering what could be wrong. He said I was to telephone Wilberforce at once, and directed me to his home across the tracks.

It was a confinement near Harcourt, Mr. Agnew told me, and would I please stay on the train and go right on. Someone would be at the crossing to meet me. Of course I said I would do so. "Why," I thought, "Did it have to be today?" This was the first time I had left town, except on "business" since September. I had been on duty 24 hours a day, seven days a week for seven straight months! Of course I was not busy all the time, but I was always on call. I didn't even know of anyone up that way who was expecting a baby. Oh well, such is life. By this time the train was ready and waiting for me. And my sister was really surprised that I had come to meet her.

The trip back did not take nearly so long as there were no long stops, but it gave us a little time to visit before we had to part at Wilberforce, where I was to carry on. I asked the conductor if they had any freight to unload there and explained the situation. I was neither dressed nor equipped to officiate at this birthday party. "You just go and take your time, Nurse. We have a little freight, but we'll wait for you." So I took time to change into my uniform and grab my bags and was back at the station just as they were finishing their business. How thankful I was for this unique I.B.&O. line! Mr. T. was waiting for me at the crossing about half a mile from his home. He carried the big suitcase and we set out walking. That time I would beat the stork by about one hour.

6

Enterprising Village Gets First Ontario Red Cross Outpost Hospital

Early history tells us that, for awhile, Wilberforce had been a thriving village with a lumber mill and several mines in operation, including mica, molybdenum, graphite and feldspar. Eventually all mineral resources in the area petered out. The community was reduced to lumbering activities, with a sawmill in the village known as the Wilberforce Lumber Company. Many families moved away, including the doctor,[1] thus leaving the community with no medical services within 25 miles and no access during the winter except by rail.

It seems incredible that a simple thing like a batch of baby chicks in an incubator could have changed that situation, but "God moves in mysterious ways, His wonders to perform" and that was the spark that set off a great nationwide movement, and it happened right here in the heart of Haliburton. The year was 1921. The Great War, fought to end all wars, was over and the little of village of Wilberforce, like other villages, was beginning to settle down to the business of living.

Many of the young men had rushed off to serve their country, several leaving wives and families to carry on as best they could. Now it was all over and the veterans, weary and some disabled, had returned

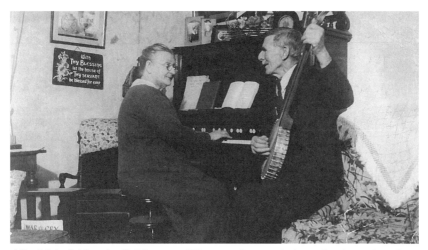

Alfred Schofield and wife Margaret (Thompson), a musical couple, shown here in their later years. They were instrumental in getting the Red Cross Outpost established in Wilberforce. *Courtesy Hilda Clark Collection.*

to their homes. Some, of course, did not return and their widows and families were struggling to get along, many in great need of care and guidance.

There had been a great wave of marriages when the veterans returned, and now the birth rate was rising rapidly. With no medical assistance available within half a day's journey, many inexperienced neighbours were called in to act as midwives or to prescribe their home remedies for various illnesses.

At that time, the Children's Aid Society Inspector for Haliburton County was Mr. Alfred G. Schofield. He and his wife had come from England several years before and for a few years had lived in Oshawa. While there, he was instrumental in founding the Oshawa General Hospital. A very benevolent couple, they were always interested in the welfare of others and always alert to any needs in the community.

When Mrs. [Margaret] Schofield's health began to fail, they moved to Wilberforce, where he performed his duties as Children's Aid Inspector for the county. For a while they lived on the Burleigh Road,[2] about two miles south of the village. Their house was situated on a steep little hill overlooking Poverty Lake,[3] with the road running past their door. It almost broke their hearts to watch the horses struggling up the hill with the sleighs loaded with heavy logs on their way to the mill, so he gave the township a strip of his level land below the hill and had them change the course of the road.

One day, in the pursuit of his work, Alfred Schofield required some information from the [Monmouth] township records, so visited the clerk, who happened to be the Methodist Minister who lived near the church at South Wilberforce. When he made his needs known, [the Reverend] Mr. Ogden got out the record books and suggested that Mr. Schofield help himself. He was very busy just then, he said, attending to some baby chicks that were hatching in his incubator. Mr. Schofield soon found out what he wanted, then continued looking through the records of births and deaths. He was shocked to see the names of so many mothers who had died at childbirth, with no doctor in attendance.

He reported his findings to the Director of the Children's Aid in Toronto, asking him to urge the government to send a maternity nurse or midwife to the county. In the reply, he was directed to write the Red Cross. Two weeks later a committee, headed by Mrs. Plumptre herself,[4] visited Wilberforce to look over the situation. They met with Mr. Schofield and other influential people of the local community on November 21, 1921, at which time Mrs. Plumptre promised the support of the Red Cross in establishing a nursing service for the community. A committee was formed and the business of securing Letters Patent, which would enable them to provide necessary accommodation, was explored. Then, in February, 1922, a nurse by the name of Miss [Josephine] Jackson[5] arrived. She took a room at the boarding house and carried on from there, travelling most of the time by horseback.

Eventually, Letters Patent were drawn up and on May 13, 1922, these were signed by Harry C. Nixon, the Provincial Secretary. The corporation was under the name of the "The Monmouth Charitable Association." The original directors were S.W. [Stanley] Reynolds, F.D. [Frank] Herlihey, J.W. [Rev. Joseph] Ogden, G.A. [Gerald] Finlay, and H.S. [Herbert] Mulloy. Incidently, at the first Annual Meeting of this Association held after my arrival, my name was added to the list of directors, which at that time included Fred Agnew, Mrs. Tom [Flora] Marshall, and H. [Harvey] Rose. Mrs. George [Eva] Barnes was President and Frank Schofield, brother of Alfred (who had moved to Haliburton in the meantime) was Secretary-Treasurer.[6]

A short time after the Letters Patent were received, an old house was purchased which was to serve for thirty-eight years as the *first Red Cross Outpost in Ontario.*

Miss Jackson was followed in 1923 by Miss [Catherine] Lawrence

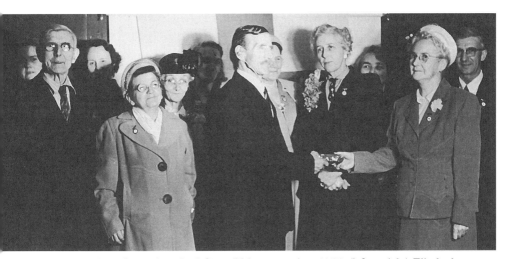

Presentation of awards to Red Cross Volunteers, circa 1955: (left to right) Elizabeth Bailey; Alfred Schofield; Nurse (Mrs.) Doris Kenny; Sophia Sanderson; Clara Schofield; Sylvia Cameron; Frank Schofield; May Croft; Evelyn Anderson; Gertrude LeRoy Miller, Viva Bowen and Jack Taylor. (The picture appears to have been taken at the Wilberforce School.) *Courtesy Wilberforce Heritage Guild.*

and, in 1924, by Miss [Anne] Casey. A year seemed about the limit of their stay, possibly because they had to work under such trying conditions without proper training.[7] The winter months with the deep snow and sub zero temperatures made their work particularly difficult. However, the project paid off in the lowering of the death rate and much suffering was relieved or prevented.

Miss [Elizabeth] Knaggs arrived in 1925 and, with her special training in midwifery in England, she was especially welcome and earned a fine reputation. After three years she was transferred to Apsley, about 35 miles in the direction of Peterborough, to open a new Outpost there. Miss [Jean Marie] Lougheed, a very conscientious nurse, but not cut out for rough country life, replaced her but stayed only a year. Likewise the nurse who replaced her did not fit in very well, and thus the telegram to me. And here I was in Wilberforce.

In the early 1920s, an old prospector with Yukon experience, Bill Richardson, lived with his wife not far from Wilberforce. He had a great faith in the hills thereabout, and took up the search, this time for pitchblende, and was successful. By 1930, when I arrived, mining activity was raising great hopes in the community. The old molybdenum mill, known many years as the "White Elephant," was being dismantled and moved to a new site and the International Radium Mine

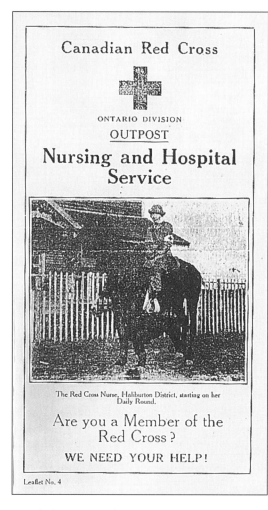

Canadian Red Cross

ONTARIO DIVISION

OUTPOST

Nursing and Hospital Service

The Red Cross Nurse, Haliburton District, starting on her Daily Round.

Are you a Member of the Red Cross?

WE NEED YOUR HELP!

Leaflet No. 4

An excerpt taken from a Red Cross pamphlet promoting community understanding of the development of a Red Cross Outpost, developed by the Ontario Division of the Canadian Red Cross Society. Josephine Jackson, the very first Red Cross Outpost nurse, is shown on horseback in front of the Wilberforce Red Cross Outpost. *Courtesy Wilberforce Heritage Guild Collection, donated by Charles Whebell, son of Josephine Jackson.*

was being opened. Later, another discovery was made at Cheddar and the Canada Radium Mine was opened there.

A townsite was built at Cheddar and mining operations carried on for awhile, but eventually they both went the way of all the other mines in the past. There was not enough ore to make them worth while. However, the International Mine did become globally famous, but not for radium. Inside the mine was a spring of sparkling clear water. Thousands of gallons were shipped all over the world because of the water's supposedly special health-giving qualities, especially with regard to fertility. I've often wondered if that might be the reason for the many very large families I encountered in that area.

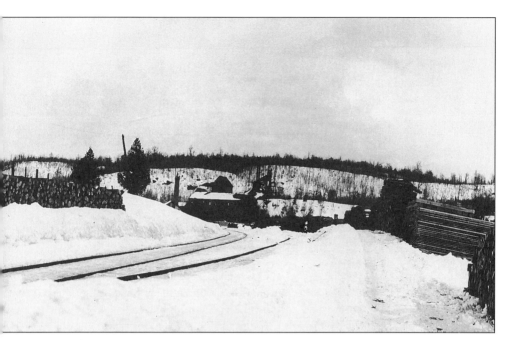

The Graphite Mine buildings, seen in the centre just beyond the I.B.& O. rail line, produced the graphite used in lead pencils. Note the great piles of cordwood and lumber piled by the siding, waiting to be shipped out by rail. *Courtesy Wilberforce Heritage Guild Collection.*

It is interesting to look over the lists of pupils who were attending the various schools in the early 1930s.[8] Many may still be living in the community and many, I'm sure, did become very prominent citizens.

When inspecting the children, I found a great many with impaired vision. There was very little hope of securing glasses if it was left to the parents. However, we were very fortunate one summer in having a Registered Optometrist vacationing at Wilbermere Farm nearby. When he learned about the situation, he made a wonderful offer. He said he would bring his equipment and examine the eyes of anyone I recommended, young or old. If he found that glasses were required, he would supply them at greatly reduced prices.

As it was summer, I arranged for him to use the Wilberforce School, and for one whole week it certainly buzzed with activity. He even supplied transportation for those who had no way of coming from out-of-town, by permitting his son to use his car for that purpose. Even at his low prices, however, many families could not afford to pay for the glasses, but he supplied them in spite of that, saying that a way would

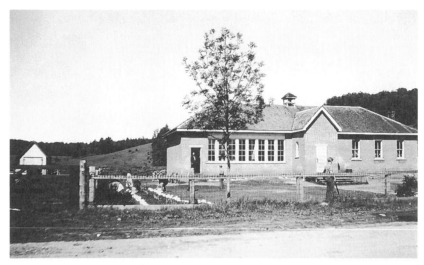

Wilberforce Consolidated Continuation School was just up the street from the Outpost, on the other side. The students seem to be gardening. That could be the teacher in the doorway. *Courtesy Agnew Family Collection.*

be found without difficulty. Shortly after I had arrived in Wilberforce, a friend in Toronto told fellow members of a Service Club (I.O.D.E.)[9] about my work and they expressed a desire to help in some way. My greatest need at that time, I felt, was a child's crib, which they supplied. Shortly after our eye clinic, I was visiting Toronto and was invited to speak at a meeting of this club. They were anxious to hear more about my work and, when I mentioned the glasses situation, they very kindly assumed the responsibility of paying the balance due on them.

Well, the eyes were looked after, for awhile. But regarding the teeth, that was another story. One could hardly blame those suffering with toothaches for calling on the village blacksmith at a nearby town, who had quite a reputation along those lines. I was told of one fellow, Josh, who had a terrible toothache so he went to see Joe, the blacksmith. Thinking it might be wise to take a bottle to fortify him against the pain of having the tooth pulled, Josh came prepared. He took a drink and gave Joe a drink, and then Joe set to work. He got out his forceps and yanked out the offending tooth and they each had another drink or two. After awhile Josh said, "My tooth still aches! You've pulled the wrong tooth!" So back went the forceps and out came another tooth, and more drinks were needed. Pretty soon Josh told Joe that he was pretty sure that he still had not pulled the right tooth, so another one came out. As this went on for some time, both men were getting quite tipsy. However, the bottle was finally empty, so Joe helped Josh out to his buggy and headed his horse toward home. The next morning when Josh woke up, he was minus all of his upper teeth! This episode happened years before my time so I cannot vouch for its accuracy. I often wondered how many teeth Josh had to begin with. However, Joe actually did pull the odd tooth, even in my time.

I also pulled a number of teeth myself, but only children's baby teeth, which were usually so loose they could have pulled them out themselves if they'd had the courage. For the time being, I could only teach oral hygiene and hope that prevention would pay off.

7

Wheels Make a Difference

I was glad to see the roads dry up near the end of April so that I could get a car of my own. It would mean that I could make many more home visits. Besides, I could come and go as I wished and the neighbours need not know everything that went on. They were the finest of neighbours, but they had little else to do for relaxation than to make sure that no one either entered or left town without their knowledge, especially if the Outpost was involved. If a team and sleigh came for me, everyone knew whose team it was and wouldn't rest until they knew who was ill and all about the situation. Even a call at night didn't go unnoticed. A neighbour suffered severely with asthma and I was called many times in the wee small hours to administer adrenalin. The next morning at least one of the neighbours would find an excuse to see me, then would eventually ask, "Did Wilf have a bad spell last night? I just happened to be up and saw you going out with your bag." When I hired someone to take me it was the same, so it would be quite a relief to have a car of my own.

I arranged to buy a new Model A Ford Coupe with a rumble seat, and judging by the various experiences I had with it, I made a wise choice. A larger car could not possibly have taken me to some of the places that it did without difficulty. Incidentally, the total cost of the car, including insurance and license, was $678.00.

My brother, Don, drove the car up from the city for me and taught

A copy of the "Bill of Sale" (1931) for Gertrude LeRoy's car, a Ford Standard Coupe with a rumble seat–complete with insurance and license. *Courtesy Gerald R. Miller and Family Collection.*

me to drive it. While I'd had lots of experience with a Model T, I knew nothing about a gearshift, but soon caught on. The next thing was to secure a driving permit, which hadn't been required before. I would have to go to Bancroft to take a test.

Most of the roads around Wilberforce, as I have already mentioned, were narrow, hilly and crooked, but none could compare with the road to Bancroft. Talk about hairpin curves! One, called "The Devil's Elbow" was well named! Another strip going up the "mountain" was just a steep narrow ledge with many curves, and with only a flimsy rail fence to prevent a sudden drop to eternity! One hill was so steep that logs had been laid across, like a corduroy road, and it was bump, bump, bump all the way up or down.

I had been over this road once since my arrival with someone else doing the driving, so at least knew what to look for. As soon as I felt sure that I could handle the car, I set out for Bancroft and, to my great relief, arrived safe and sound. When the man who was to give me the test got in the car, he asked me if I had driven all the way from Wilberforce myself. When I assured him that I had he said, "Well, I guess you certainly must know how to drive."

Soon I was not afraid to go anywhere and it was not long until nearly everyone in the country knew the little maroon car, and knew when the nurse was in the community. Often they would be waiting to catch me on the way back to town, perhaps to ask my advice or to have me call in to see someone who was ill, or even to send a message to someone along the way. I discovered a case of Polio in that way. A mother saw me pass on my way to the nearby school and sent a little tot with a note asking me to stop in on my way back. Her little boy was quite sick. They had taken him to the doctor several days ago, but he hadn't responded to the medicine and was much worse. As soon as I saw him, I suspected Polio: a stiff neck, weak legs, high temperature... All of these symptoms had developed since the visit to the doctor. Acting on my advice, they sent for a doctor immediately and when he saw the child, he confirmed my suspicions. I am thankful to say that the child made a complete recovery.

One evening, a man appeared at the door and asked me to come and look after his wife who was having her first baby. He had walked from South Monmouth, some fifteen miles away. If he hadn't been with me, I would never have found his home. We had to travel about seven miles along the main road, then about the same distance or more off onto a less travelled sideroad without passing a single habitation. At last he said, "Here we are. Turn left."

"Is this a road?" I asked. "Can we drive through here?" I had to strain my eyes to see wagon tracks leading into the thick bush.

"Oh, yes. It's level and dry," was the answer. "Other cars have been in."

Well, it was level and dry all right, but barely wide enough to get through. It was as if we were driving through a small tunnel. To make matters worse, we hadn't gone very far when whom should we come upon but "Mr. Porcupine," travelling in the same direction only at a much slower pace. Even several blasts of the horn would not persuade him to allow intruders into his domain. My passenger finally got out and, breaking a small branch off a tree finally induced him, with a few strong proddings, to jog to the left and let us pass. Who but a porcupine would want to live in such a place anyway?

At last we reached a bit of a clearing with a rough tarpaper shack and a couple other similar buildings. Finding the patient in the second stage of labour, I had to work fast. I was thankful for my suitcase[1] full of supplies for there was practically nothing to work with in the home.

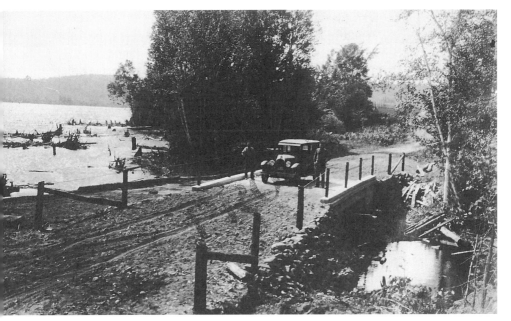

A scenic postcard view of an early-model car on an early road, said to be at Richardson's Bridge, Wilberforce. *Courtesy Wilberforce Heritage Guild Collection.*

Her nearest neighbour from a mile or so away was with her. She had a good fire on and a big pot of boiling water on the stove. In general, the place was neat and tidy, although sparse.

I was glad of the neighbour's help and, before long, another miracle had taken place. A healthy baby boy was born and the mother was well and happy. Knowing it would be impossible for me to return daily to care for them, I left instructions and some supplies with my helper, who said she could stay for a few days. After ensuring that all was well, I took off.

I was not worried about losing my way, as there was only one path that I could see, but I was heartbroken the next day when I saw all the scratches on my new car! On my way home I had wondered why a man would take his wife to such an isolated spot to live and raise a family. I was sure he wasn't even pretending to do any farming. Later, however, I learned that there was quite a bit of moonshine being made in that vicinity.

A few days following I admitted a patient who was in her mid 40s and expecting her tenth child. I was very concerned about her and was finally successful in persuading her husband that she must have a doctor. He did have Mr. Agnew call Dr. Frain.[2] It was a very complicated case, which required every ounce of his skill and strength to deliver her. As I was giving the anesthetic, I asked if there was anything else I could do. "Yes," he said, "Pray." Indeed I had been doing that ever since labour began.

The mother survived but the baby did not. What if I had been alone with her? Another prayer was given for the presence of Dr. Frain and his skill and for the fact that I had been able to help in saving her life. It could so easily have been two lives lost. Having her at the Outpost for two weeks of good care in a quiet friendly environment did wonders for her both physically and emotionally.

It wasn't quiet for long though because, two days after her delivery, another patient arrived. I heard a car stop and when I reached the front door, there stood a rickety old touring car. A young man was trying to help his passenger out. She was a big woman, judged to be in her 20s, with a quilt wrapped around her. I could tell she was in great pain. "What's wrong?" I asked, hurrying out to help. "She's been burned," the man replied.

Between us we managed to get her into the building and up the narrow stairway. Aileen had gone ahead and had the bed turned down. What a pity we had only one bed downstairs! The man, her brother, told us what had happened. His sister was housecleaning and had taken an iron bed outside and was washing it with what he thought was water, from a pail nearby. He had come along and, finishing a cigarette, had tossed it into the pail. It wasn't water. It was gasoline!

As soon as we got her onto the bed, I sent him to the store to get Mr. Agnew to call a doctor, and to tell him exactly what had happened so he could come prepared. In the meantime, I took it upon myself to give her a shot of morphine to lessen her suffering. I was horrified to find that she was burned literally from head to toe. Being a big fleshy person, that comprised a very large area. With Aileen helping me, we managed to remove her clothing and I cleaned the burned area as well as I could. I didn't know what treatment the doctor would use, but thought he might want to spray the area with tannic acid, the latest treatment I had seen used for burns. I prepared a solution of it and filled an atomizer to be ready when he arrived. When sprayed over a burned area, tannic acid forms an astringent coating.

Fortunately, Dr. Frain was available and arrived in record time, bringing with him a solution of tannic acid and an atomizer. Between us, we soon had the burned areas all covered. Part of her face, chest and abdomen, and one leg from hip to instep were the most severely burned. Dr. Frain left orders regarding the changing of her dressings and also instructed that she have morphine when necessary. And it certainly was necessary many times, especially when the dressings were changed. He saw her just that one time, but by following his orders and using my utmost skill, under the direction of the Great Physician, I was very thankful to be able to discharge her, completely healed, in three weeks.

Four days after admitting the burned patient, Dr. Speck arrived with another patient, a woman who was hemorrhaging. She was having a miscarriage, he said. Whether or not she had induced it herself he didn't know, but he would have to operate to stop the bleeding.

An emergency operation here? With a maternity patient downstairs and a burn patient upstairs? Only Aileen's bed and mine were left! I would just have to turn my room into an operating room with no time to waste. Fortunately, my predecessor[3] happened to be visiting friends in town, so I sent Aileen to see if she would give us a hand. Dr. Speck gave me what instruments he had, and I gathered up ours and put

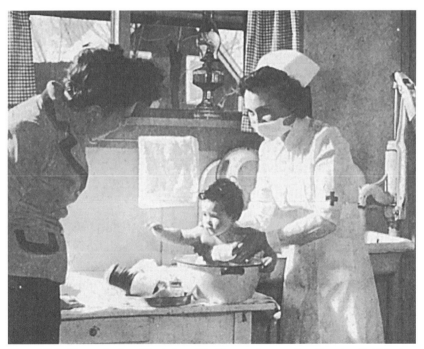

Nurse Elsie Turner bathes Gloria Jane Herlihey, as her mother Beatrice (Schicker) Herlihey watches, circa 1940s. *Courtesy Wilberforce Heritage Guild Collection.*

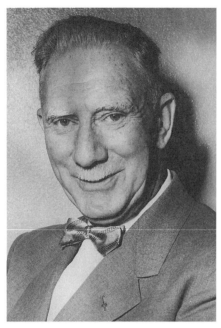

Dr. John Speck, a highly-respected medical doctor served in Haliburton and area while Gertrude LeRoy was at the Outpost. She would have often worked with him. Dr. Speck left the area in 1941 and went, with his family, including twin sons Bill and Jack, to Cooksville where he was the coroner for a time. He died about 1970. *Courtesy William J. Speck, son of Dr. J. Speck.*

them all on to boil. There were plenty of sterile sheets, towels, gowns, gloves, and dressings on hand so by the time the instruments were sterilized, we had everything set up and the patient prepared. Dr. Speck anesthetized the patient, then turned that part over to the other nurse and I scrubbed up and assisted the doctor. Everything worked out very successfully.

Well, now we had three patients. I wondered what the other nurse was thinking. She had been here for nearly a year with "nothing to do."

I had to keep in mind that burn cases anywhere near a maternity patient or a gynecological case requires the utmost caution in aseptic techniques. These patients can easily be infected with germs causing blood poison, which in those days before the development of antibiotics, often proved fatal. Fortunately, all of our patients were discharged healthy and strong, without a second visit from the doctors. Of course, we had the Great Physician watching over us.

We had one day that June without a patient. I do not recall what we did to celebrate, but the next day an unexpected maternity patient arrived. Fortunately, she had arranged to have a doctor so I was relieved of much of the responsibility. Aileen and I were both happy to have a wee baby to look after, but this wee one was just two days old when Dr. Speck arrived with a little one-year-old girl from a small village a few miles beyond Haliburton, completely outside my territory. He said she was in desperate need of good nursing care and he was sure I would take her in. Poor child! How could I refuse? Our hearts ached for her. Practically her whole body was covered with a

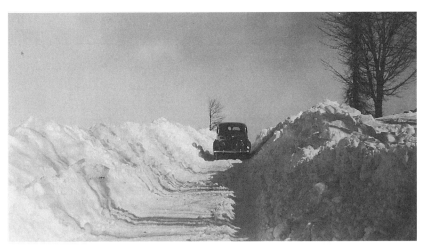

During the winter of 1937–38, Dr. Speck took a picture of his 1937 Ford, showing the height of the snowbanks. *Courtesy William J. Speck, son of Dr. J. Speck.*

rash, eczema he said. He told us she was from a large poverty-stricken family and her mother was unable to cope with the situation.

How fortunate it was that I had suggested a child's crib rather than a bassinet when the I.O.D.E. group offered to send us some equipment. The crib had often been divided to serve as two or three bassinets. Now, when little Dorothy arrived we were ready for her. On warm sunny days we moved the crib out onto the lawn, and with good nourishing meals, proper treatment and tender loving care the child began a wonderful recovery.

In the meantime, I had been informed that I had been chosen to go to New York to observe several Public Health programs in action. Two of us were to go (drive) and we would spend one week at Olean[4] observing the Cattaraugus County Health Demonstration, about which we had recently studied at university. Then to New York City's Maternity Center and Henry Street Mission. We would leave July 1st.

I have already mentioned the need for dental care in the community, so needless to say I was delighted when I learned that the Ontario Department of Health would loan us a dentist for a month during the summer. He would set up his equipment in a room at the Outpost and treat anyone requiring his services free of charge. Unfortunately, he would not arrive until after my departure for New York. But fortunately, the nurse who was to relieve me was well known to me from training days, and I knew she would be quite capable of handling the situation.

Every summer the local Red Cross held a big community picnic for

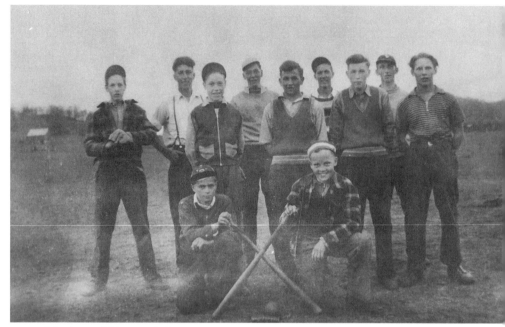

Members of this 1938 ball team, the photograph taken in Minden, Ontario, were also known to play at Red Cross picnic games. Back row: (left to right) Bill Riley, Hugh Perry, Murray Agnew, Ernie Tallman, Jim Miller. Middle row: Glen Johnston, Albert Sanderson, Ken Sanderson, David Croft. Front row: Bill Elliott, Royce Godfrey. *Courtesy Agnew Family Collection.*

the purpose of raising money for the upkeep of the Outpost. Committees would work for weeks making plans and preparations. The main features of the afternoon would be a ball game between our team and one from outside, speeches by local members of both Provincial and Federal governments, as well as various other officials, usually someone from Red Cross Headquarters [in Toronto]. There were also games and races for anyone choosing to do so, and ice cream cones and pop. As well, Red Cross tags[5] would be on sale throughout the day.

At suppertime the doors of the Orange Hall would be thrown open revealing long tables groaning under loads of delicious food. During the last two weeks or so the food committee would have canvassed the whole district for food. The response was always so tremendous: pies of all kinds, homemade bread, butter, pickles, vegetables, salads, cakes,…Many would give money that would be used to buy meat, tea and other baked goods requiring purchase. Most of the local women would be on hand and each would have a job, filling plates, waiting

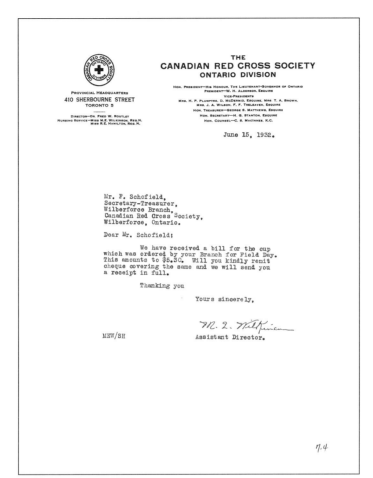

THE
CANADIAN RED CROSS SOCIETY
ONTARIO DIVISION

HON. PRESIDENT—HIS HONOUR, THE LIEUTENANT-GOVERNOR OF ONTARIO
PRESIDENT—W. H. ALDERSON, ESQUIRE
VICE-PRESIDENTS
MRS. H. P. PLUMPTRE, D. McDERMID, ESQUIRE, MRS. T. A. BROWN,
MRS. J. A. WILSON, F. F. TRELEAVEN, ESQUIRE
HON. TREASURER—GEORGE S. MATTHEWS, ESQUIRE
HON. SECRETARY—H. G. STANTON, ESQUIRE
HON. COUNSEL—C. S. MacINNES, K.C.

PROVINCIAL HEADQUARTERS
410 SHERBOURNE STREET
TORONTO 5

DIRECTOR—DR. FRED W. ROUTLEY
NURSING SERVICE—MISS M.E. WILKINSON, REG.N.
MISS R.E. HAMILTON, REG. N.

June 15, 1932.

Mr. F. Schofield,
Secretary-Treasurer,
Wilberforce Branch,
Canadian Red Cross Society,
Wilberforce, Ontario.

Dear Mr. Schofield:

We have received a bill for the cup
which was ordered by your Branch for Field Day.
This amounts to $5.30. Will you kindly remit
cheque covering the same and we will send you
a receipt in full.

Thanking you

Yours sincerely,

M. E. Wilkinson
Assistant Director.

MEW/SH

7.4

Letter to Frank Schofield, June 1932, requesting payment for the trophy cup to be awarded at the annual Red Cross picnic. *Courtesy Wilberforce Heritage Guild Collection.*

on tables, or washing dishes. As soon as the last person was fed, the tables would be cleared and removed to their storage place, chairs and benches lined up along the walls and the floor swept, to be made ready for the dance which was to follow. During the afternoon another group of women would be busy at the Outpost preparing sandwiches to be served at the dance.

No one would think of missing the Red Cross picnic. It was the one big outing of the year and, if for no other reason, some would come to see friends whom they had not seen since the previous picnic. Many a cow was not milked until very late that night. Those who lived nearby could go home and do their chores and return for the dance. But, since not many had cars, they just stayed on.

This year as usual, the picnic was scheduled for July 1st, just three days before I was to leave for Toronto. To complicate matters, we still had our little Dorothy at the Outpost, which meant that one of us would have to be there to look after her, so we would take turns. Fortunately, both the hall and the school grounds where all the activities were taking place were not far away, and the relief nurse was expected to arrive on the train about suppertime.

At last July 1st dawned, bright and hot; 98 degrees in the shade during the afternoon, someone said. A big ball game was in progess between the local and Bancroft teams and, by the sound of the cheering, the local team was doing well. I was on my way to the hall when whom should I meet but my brother,[6] and not far behind were my mother[7] and Beulah Scott, the nurse who was to relieve me!

Miss Scott had trained with me and, when she had learned that she was to relieve me, she called to tell my mother. Don, always looking for an excuse to come to Wilberforce, offered to drive her and mother up in time for the picnic and surprise me. They had to return early the next morning, so Beulah and I had two whole days together before my departure Saturday morning. Needless to say, we had a lot to talk about besides the duties of a Red Cross Nurse.

As I had not spent a summer here myself, it was difficult to predict what the next five weeks would bring forth, but I certainly did not tell her she would have nothing to do. At least it was more like a hospital than when I arrived.

8

Poverty and the Deepening Depression

While I was away, for some reason or other, business slackened up considerably. Miss Scott had assisted a doctor at a home confinement and had discharged our little eczema patient, but outside of that she said there wasn't much to report. The dentist had arrived and set up his equipment in one of the rooms and was doing a rushing business.

I was home only a short time, however, when my work picked up with a vengeance. Aileen and I were quietly eating our supper one evening when Mr. Agnew came with a message from Gooderham. A little girl had come to the station and asked the agent to call the nurse as her mother was sick. He had no other information except that they lived about two miles past the village in a log house. It could be a confinement I thought, so I should go prepared for that. If so, I could not expect to get back until long after dark, and I was not keen about a 20 mile drive on a lonely road by myself late at night. In fact, Miss Hamilton [1] had made me promise to always take someone with me if possible under such circumstances. What if I should have a flat tire (quite common in those days) or other car trouble?

So, while I was gathering my things together, Aileen went down to see if Hazel Miller, Del's sister, would go with me. She had finished

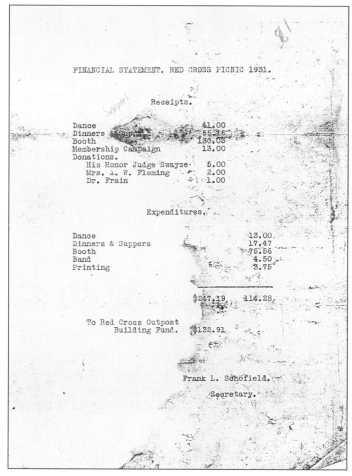

FINANCIAL STATEMENT. RED CROSS PICNIC 1931.

Receipts.

Dance	41.00
Dinners	55.15
Booth	130.03
Membership Campaign	13.00

Donations.

His Honor Judge Swayze	5.00
Mrs. A. W. Fleming	2.00
Dr. Frain	1.00

Expenditures.

Dance	13.00
Dinners & Suppers	17.47
Booth	75.56
Band	4.50
Printing	3.75

$247.19   114.28

To Red Cross Outpost
Building Fund. $132.91

Frank L. Schofield.

Secretary.

A reproduction of the Wilberforce Red Cross picnic "Financial Statement," 1931. *Courtesy Wilberforce Heritage Guild Collection.*

her course at Normal School and was home for the summer. Together we set out and finally found the house which I was sure must be the right one. I had often passed it and noticed its dilapidated condition and could hardly believe that anyone lived there.

A tall, thin, untidy-looking man and four very dirty children stood around the open doorway as I drove up. Hazel stayed in the car and, as I walked up the path, the children disappeared. The father led the way into a fairly large kitchen, which was swarming with flies. The table was littered with dirty dishes, bread crusts and other debris, and the floor needed a good sweeping.

Two doors led off to the left. The first one was open and revealed the patient, lying on a bare filthy mattress and covered with a once-white flannelette sheet. Her pillow, minus a cover. was very dirty as well. "Good evening Mrs. R.," I said. "I got your message to come. Are you having a baby?"

"Yes, Nurse. I sent for you as soon as the pains started but they still ain't comin very fast."

"Well, that's good," I replied. "That will give us time to get cleaned up a bit. Is it coming ahead of time?"

"No, I figure it's about time."

After checking her physical condition and assuring her that everything seemed normal, I set to work. Fortunately, there was enough warm water on the stove for me to give her a good cleansing bath and I asked her husband to put more on to heat. I was glad that my bag produced a couple of extra sheets and a pillowcase, for she said she had none except what was on the bed. As well, the dirty old house-dress she was wearing needed replacing. In the bag also were hospital gowns, towels, washcloths, soap, a large rubber sheet and a layette for the baby, if needed.

At last I had her prepared for delivery and the bed made up except for the sterile supplies which would be opened later. While making up the room, I remembered a remark that Dr. S.S. Lumb[2] made while I was assisting him at a home delivery, "I would much rather deliver patients in their own homes because they are immune to their own germs." Personally, I prefer the hospital.

Most expectant mothers I had come into contact with took great pride in preparing for the new baby, whether it was number one or number ten, even if some of the articles had already seen much use. When I asked this mother, however, where I might find things for her baby, she said, "I really haven't had time to get anything ready, Nurse."

"Haven't you any pieces of soft cloth or old diapers, or anything we could use to wrap the baby in?" I asked.

"Just look in those drawers, Nurse, you might find something that will do."

There was a large chest of drawers and also a beautiful china cabinet in the bedroom, so out of keeping with the rest of the surroundings. Even the bed she was lying in had, at one time been a beautiful brass bed, I'm sure. These people must have known better times, at least the furniture had.

I opened one drawer after another but could find nothing but a jumble of dirty rags. Even the shelves of the china cabinet were stuffed with old clothing, nothing clean enough to wrap around a new baby. Bless the women throughout Canada who sew for the Red Cross! This baby would have a new layette from my suitcase!

I emptied one of the drawers and transformed it into a bassinet, then decided to have a little rest. In the meantime, Hazel had come in and was helping the husband tidy up the kitchen. The children had been sent to bed.

Mr. R. offered to make a place for us to lie down in the "other room." Of course we had no intention of doing that, but just for curiosity I went with him to see where he intended to put us. I still don't know for there was just one bed, and it already had four sleeping children in it. We went out and sat in the car for awhile and about two hours later the baby arrived, a normal delivery with no problems.

It was just breaking day when we started for home. As there was no one except the husband to care for them, I felt it was necessary to return every day while the patient was in bed. At least she and the baby were kept clean for ten days.

Incidentally, I received a letter about a year later from this woman saying she was expecting another baby in about two weeks and would like me to come and take care of her again. So far, she said, she had not had time to get anything ready, but would try to get some things for the baby in time. Through the grapevine I learned that there had been no time to get anyone except her nearest neighbour. No preparations had been made so the neighbours donated clothing.

It would soon be a year since my arrival at Wilberforce and, although I was much better prepared for the new school year, I had learned that the activities of Mr. Stork took priority over most others.

Since one of the tasks of the School Inspector was the placing of new recruits in suitable schools in his inspectorate, Hazel was sent to Kennaway,[3] an isolated hamlet about fifteen miles to the north. This was one of the oldest settlements in the district and had once been quite a hive of activity, including having a sawmill. Now, however, only four families remained, scattered over an area of about two miles. Those who were left made their living, such as it was, by working their farms, though no one would hardly recognize them as such, and trapping. Fish and game were quite plentiful, which helped keep them from starving during those early 1930s when times were really lean.

Hazel boarded at the home of the secretary of the school board and had about half a mile to walk to school. (Once she met a bear on the

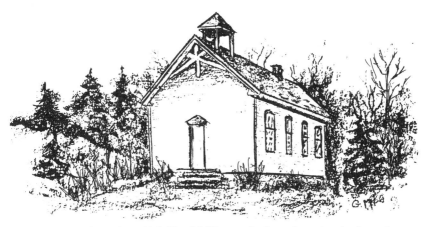

The Kennaway School at which Hazel Miller taught for a short time in the early 1930s, a school well-surrounded by forest. Original sketch by Gertrude LeRoy Miller.

road and was so frightened she didn't know what to do. She stopped and looked at the bear, then turned around and walked away. The bear did the same, in the opposite direction!) There were nine children on the roll, ranging in age from six to sixteen. Often I would drive in for her on a Friday afternoon and take her back Sunday evening.

One Friday while I was waiting at the school for her, a neighbour came to see me. She told me she was expecting a baby in about a month and would like to make arrangements to have it at the Outpost. I asked all the questions I would have in a regular pre-natal visit and decided she was all right. Two weeks later I stopped in to see her and suggested that she be prepared to come out with me the next week when I brought Hazel back. This would give her at least a week in Wilberforce before her baby was born, which would be much better than waiting until the last minute. She had no means of transportation other than horseback, and no means of calling me, but had friends in town where she could stay. This would be her sixth child, so she would not likely be long in labor. While I had two patients at the Outpost, at least one was expected to be discharged by that time.

Well, the next morning I awoke with the strangest feeling. Something told me that I should go after Mrs. C. that day and not even wait until I had taken Hazel back Sunday. I could not get her off my mind all morning. Still, I had my patients to care for and a couple of calls to make. When I was free, about three o'clock, I decided to drive out to see her at least. I stopped in at the boarding house to see if Miss

91

Taylor and Miss Chambers would like to go for the ride. I felt so strongly about the patient that I put the big suitcase and black bag into the car in case I might need them.

When she greeted me at the door she said she had never been so glad to see anyone before. At about two o'clock she'd had her first warning that her time was near. Her husband was away in the bush and she was about to send one of the children for her neighbour. She was not actually having any pains, but was sure they would be starting soon. As her husband turned up just then, so she wasted no time getting ready to come with us.

I couldn't help but think of what a wonderful change it would be for her to spend ten days at the Outpost, for her home was absolutely bare of any comforts. To begin with, there wasn't a pane of glass in any of the windows. Of course the weather was warm then, but I wondered what they did when it got cold and stormy. There was one large room downstairs which served as kitchen and bedroom. It contained a cookstove, a large table, a long bench, one kitchen chair and a rocking chair. As well, there were several large blocks of wood which, no doubt, were used as chairs, and in one corner was a battered iron bed. An open stairway, almost as steep as a ladder, led to the second floor. The children were all clean but had very little on; all were barefoot. Mrs. C. herself had on a faded print dress and canvass shoes with no stockings. Despite the obvious poverty, the whole place was clean and tidy.

My other passengers had climbed into the rumble seat along with the bags and, as soon as Mrs. C. got settled in front, we started off. I drove as carefully as I could, not wanting anything to happen on the way. Much of the trip was like going through the wilderness, for we wouldn't pass a house in ten miles.

Mrs. C. stood the trip very well, without a single pain, so we enjoyed the supper Aileen had waiting for us. Since the only bed I could give this patient was my own, after supper I made it up for her. It seemed prudent to complete all preparation for her delivery just in case I might not have time later. As she decided to have a rest, I left a bell with her and went down to do some work on my records. By that time visitors were arriving for the other patients, one upstairs and one down. The train had come in and Aileen had gone down to get the mail. I just nicely sat down at my desk when I heard Mrs. C.'s bell.

Well, the next thirty minutes were busy ones! I was lucky to have everything ready. When Aileen returned, I sent her to look into the crib. We had a baby doll which we used in the Home Nursing classes

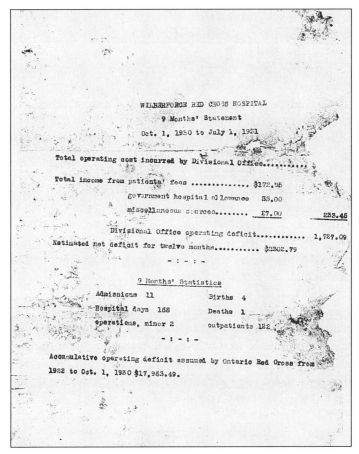

WILBERFORCE RED CROSS HOSPITAL

9 Months' Statement

Oct. 1, 1930 to July 1, 1931

Total operating cost incurred by Divisional Office........

Total income from patients' fees $172.95

        government hospital allowance   33.00

        miscellaneous sources......... 27.00   233.45

      Divisional Office operating deficit............ 1,727.09

Estimated net deficit for twelve months........... $2302.79

      - : - : -

9 Months' Statistics

Admissions 11   Births 4

Hospital days 168   Deaths 1

Operations, minor 2   outpatients 122

      - : - : -

Accumulative operating deficit assumed by Ontario Red Cross from 1922 to Oct. 1, 1930 $17,963.49.

A reproduction of the "9 Months' Statement" (October 1, 1930–July 1, 1931), likely prepared by Frank Schofield as Treasurer. *Courtesy Wilberforce Heritage Guild Collection.*

and Aileen thought I was playing a joke on her, until she took a closer look. Everything happened so quickly and so quietly that the other patients and their visitors did not know there was anything going on until they heard the baby cry.

Mrs. C. was an exceptional patient. We enjoyed every minute of the time she was there. One would never dream that she came from such an austere home. And we could not understand why her home should be that way for she was bright, talented and full of energy and good humor. She could knit, crochet and embroider beautifully, and kept us busy providing materials for her to work on in order to keep her in bed.

One very cold afternoon that fall when I was called to one of her neighbours, Mrs. C. was with her. While I was there she hurried home and returned with a pair of woollen mittens. She said she had knit them for me. She said she was sure my hands must get cold while driving. (No heaters in the cars in those days). The following fall Mrs. C. visited the Outpost for the second time, to give birth to her seventh child. Although her arrival was not as dramatic as the first, we did enjoy her stay.

I had been in Wilberforce a little more than a year when something happened which brought me to my senses. To say the least, this first year as Red Cross Nurse had certainly been eventful beyond my wildest dreams. I had arrived a complete stranger and had plunged into the work with great enthusiasm, confident that it was the will of God and that He would guide and strengthen me in my efforts. Now I was becoming overwhelmed by the immensity of the job in its many aspects. First of all was the great responsibility resting on my shoulders of the lives of the mothers who were depending on me to deliver them. Added to that was the education of the families regarding the need for immunization against communicable diseases and the getting it done, and the need of better health services for the school children, especially those regarding their teeth and eyes. As a result of my experiences in Olean and New York, I realized how much more should and could be done, but was finding that very few of the local people were as enthusiastic as I was. They knew very little of what was going on in the outside world and cared less. What was good enough for their parents was good enough for them. Why all these new fangled ideas? I was becoming very frustrated and began to feel that perhaps I was not capable of handling this job.

A long talk with Dr. Frain about my feelings didn't really help. "When I came up to this country," he said, "I, like you, was going to reform the whole district. But I soon found out that it couldn't be done, so I decided to do my job as a physician, heal the sick and let it go at that."

Well, that was all right for him, but I was a Public Health Nurse whose aim was not only to care for the sick, but the prevention of disease and the promotion of health. In carrying out these duties, it was often necessary for me to take on the functions of a social worker as well.

By now, I had visited most of my twelve schools twice and whereas during the nine years the Outpost had been open before my arrival there were 40 hospital days recorded, I had, to date, 230 and I'd had the responsibility of ten confinements alone. So I guess I was just a bit tired.

Del came to call one evening when I was alone and found me very depressed. This job was too big for me I told him. I wasn't capable of handling it so I might as well give up. I must have been in a real state, certainly in no mood for company, but it did give me a chance to air all my troubles. He just let me rave on for a while then quietly went over to the bookshelves.

"I'll tell you what I do whenever I feel that way," he said as he picked up the Bible and opened it at Psalm 23. "Let's read this." We read it together, even though we both knew every word by heart. Then I broke down and cried, and cried. Hadn't I been foolish! Here I was trying to carry all these burdens on my own strength until it had run out. I had been too "busy" to remember where to look for guidance and strength and I hadn't realized that so many changes require time and patience. Here was the answer. To think that I had come here to help these people and one of them was helping me! Now I felt strengthened and ready to carry on.

9

Ingenuity Keeps the Wolf
From Most Doors

L iving among the inhabitants of this isolated community, I began
to learn a great deal about their way of life. The sawmill in town
had been sold[1] and moved away just pior to my arrival, so the men
had to seek employment elsewhere. Many found winter work in
nearby logging camps but during other seasons had to travel far to
other mills. Most of the surrounding farms were on poor stony ground
that produced less than a decent living. Usually each had a small herd
of cattle that pastured in the fields and woods during the summer and
nearly starved during the winter, as there was often not enough good
hay grown to feed them. Many of the farmers drew marsh hay, which
grew wild on the marshes, sometimes miles from home. This had
much less food value than the hay grown on their farms, but it was
free for the cutting and drawing home. As they usually had to travel
several miles, they would camp on the spot until the job was finished.
All hay had to be cut with scythes and raked by hand because of the
swampy condition of the ground.

The only heating fuel was wood, so a good supply was necessary
for both heating and cooking. Early in the fall the men would cut what
wood they thought ought to see their families through the winter, then
take off for the camp, leaving their wives and children to look after

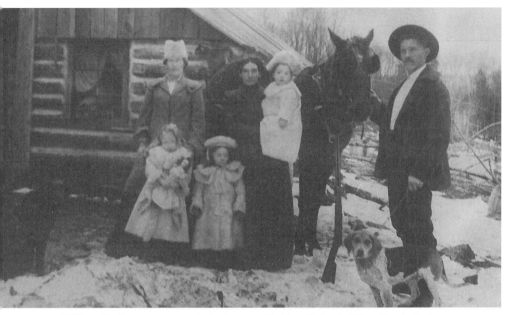

William R. Curry, camp cook, is shown with his wife Jessie Ellen (Barr), their daughter, Ethel, and son, Ronald. To the left is Mrs. McPhadden, with her daughter, Linetta. Both W.R. Curry and his wife were born in Irondale and moved to Tory Hill in 1904. After two years in that community, the family moved to Haliburton where he purchased a livery stable and lumbering business. Later, this enterprise would develop into an automobile dealership. *Courtesy Wilberforce Heritage Guild Collection.*

themselves and the stock. If their horses could be used at the camp they took them, which would lessen the responsibility for the family. If the camp was fairly close, they came home every Saturday night and returned Sunday afternoon. They usually got a few days off at Christmas, then not again until the thaw or spring breakup sometime in March or April.

Camp life, I was told, was anything but pleasant, especially the conditions under which the men had to work. About September, the first thing done was to build the camp, usually at wherever it would be convenient to the working area, usually a temporary affair to be used only one or two winters. If built of logs, it would be fairly comfortable, but that type was expensive so most were built of lumber, a single wall covered with tarpaper. There would be about fifty men to a camp, so double bunks, two tiers high, were built around the walls. These had no springs or mattresses, just bare boards with marsh hay thrown on or, lacking that, baled hay would be used. Blankets com-

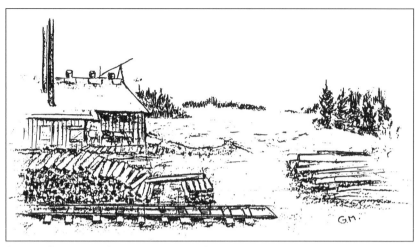

Sketch of the Wilberforce Lumber Mill. Original work by Gertrude LeRoy Miller.

pleted the bed, and anyone wanting a pillow brought his own from home.

A large barrel stove that would take four-foot chunks of wood would be set up in the middle or, if the camp were extra large, there would be one at each end. All around the stove the men would hang "Christmas trees." These were hooked sticks with spikes driven in to serve as racks for hanging all their rigging to dry, articles such as socks, insoles, mitts, rubbers…A roaring hot fire would be kept going in the stove and, by the time everybody went to bed, there would be a terrific heat. That, combined with the odours from various items hanging on the "Christmas trees," plus the sweat pads, lines and other harness pieces which the teamsters brought in to dry out, made the air almost suffocating, especially for those sleeping in the top bunks.

The men never saw the camp in daylight except on Sunday. When they were cutting the logs they worked right through the daylight hours, using all of them, but when the haul started they would have to start earlier in order to get the lead team off. Lights (coal oil lamps) always had to be out by nine o'clock at night. Sometimes the boss would turn the clock ahead an hour in order to get the men out an hour earlier in the morning. The men used to say that the boss liked them so well that he would get them up in the middle of the night to give them something to eat.

Before the haul could start, the roads would have to be prepared, first of all by plowing. Two or three teams would be hitched to a V

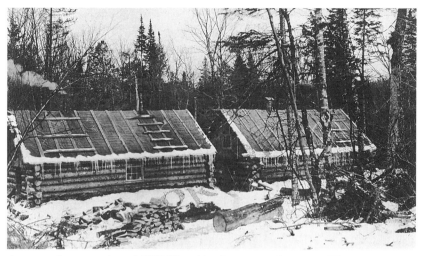

A postcard presentation of Alf Willows' lumber camp, circa 1925. He was married to Aileen Ames' sister Phyllis. *Courtesy Wilberforce Heritage Guild Collection.*

plow, a large wooden wedge affair, and drawn along the road, taking hours to go a mile or so depending on the depth of the snow. These roads would extend for miles through the bush and across the frozen lakes to the mill. Then the roads would have to be tanked. They drew large tanks of water, which they poured along the runner tracks to freeze. The horses would be sharp shod to keep them from slipping. The hills up and down which the logs had to be drawn, were kept sanded with burned sand[2] and the gangs that looked after that part of the operation were called "sandpipers." If there came a snowstorm during the night, the sandpipers would have to go out with torches to prepare the hill before the first sleighload of logs came along.

The food supplies for the camp were brought in by a cadge (hauling sleigh) team. If it were a long haul, there would be a team kept on purpose for hauling supplies, sometimes making only one trip in four days, stopping over at a halfway place. Often the way they got their meat was "on the hoof." They would drive several heads of cattle into the camp in the fall, feed them well and slaughter them as needed. Most camps kept pigs and fed them on the refuse from the cookery. The pigs were killed as pork was needed for food.

Every Saturday night was concert night for those who stayed in camp. They would sing folk songs; some were very fine singers. Some would recite poetry, particularly the poems of Robert Service. Paul Bunyan stories were told quite frequently too, as well as personal stories out of their own experiences. These, naturally, would often be made as fantastic as imagination would allow.

Yes, life in the logging camp must have been quite a life, and all for the grand sum of thirty-five to forty dollars a month plus board! Some men made extra money by trapping, and many made that their main vocation. A fair variety of fur-bearing animals, though not very plentiful, included beaver, mink, muskrats, red fox, weasles, some otter and the odd fisher. Pelts were sold to fur buyers who travelled through the country, offering as little money as possible. For pelts that were well put up, the approximate prices at that time were: beaver $10 to $15; mink $5 to $10; muskrat $2; fox $15; weasel $1; otter $15 to $20. Anyone lucky enough to get a small dark female fisher might get as high as $65. When the logging camps closed in the spring, life still had to go on.

My education expanded in many areas besides nursing during that first year or so in this great wilderness. I learned that in a place like this the local people must depend upon nature and hard work to provide most of their food. It was therefore very enlightening for me to take part in the search for variety in that way, rather than just buy everything at the store.

Early one spring I was introduced to the art of making maple syrup. Mr. [George] Miller had the use of a sugar bush a mile or so down the road, so one beautiful day Mrs. [Melissa] Miller, Mrs. [Flora] Marshall and I decided to walk down and see what was going on. Mr. Miller was gathering the sap in pails and carrying it to the boiling place, where he had three huge iron pots hanging by chains from a pole supported at each end by crotched poles. A fire was kept burning furiously under the kettles. The sap was poured into the first kettle and, as it boiled down, it was dipped into the next one, then into the third. This one was for finishing off the sap and had to be watched very carefully. We were told that forty gallons of sap had to be boiled down to make one gallon of syrup.

To tap a tree, a hole is bored into the trunk of a maple tree and a spile driven in. A spile is really a spout that catches the sap as it rises up the trunk. In the early days these were made of wood, whittled out by hand. Mr. Miller made a few of these when he ran out of the metal ones. The sap buckets, hung onto these, catch the clear sparkling sap as drop by drop it splashes into the receptacle. It has the appearance of clear water but tastes slightly sweet.

The weather has a great deal to do with the flow of sap. Cold frosty

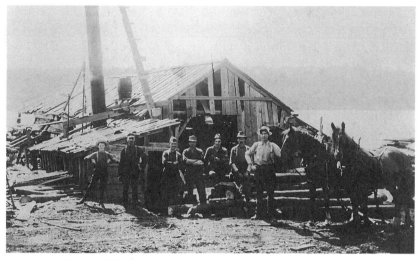

A pause at Finlay's Mill, the photograph taken circa 1915. This mill would be demolished by fire in 1920. *Courtesy Wilberforce Heritage Guild Collection.*

nights and warm sunny days are ideal. As the sap boils it turns a light amber colour, and the longer it boils the darker and thicker it gets. Great care must be taken to start to "sugar off" before it gets too thick and burns. A small piece of fat pork will keep it from boiling over. As the time comes for the actual sugaring off, the fire is allowed to die down and the syrup is tested every few minutes by letting some run off the edge of the dipper. When the final drops run together just so, it is ready. The syrup then is strained through a cotton bag into a cream can and taken home to be finished.

I watched the finishing process at the house as well. The syrup was put on the stove in large kettles and heated. Milk and egg [whites] were added to clarify it and it was boiled and skimmed, and boiled and skimmed, until the proper thickness was attained. It then was strained through another bag and bottled for future use. And was it ever good!

Making maple syrup was certainly a lot of work, especially in those days (methods have advanced considerably since then), but everyone seemed to enjoy it. Once the flow of sap slacken and growth starts in the trees, it's time to pull the spiles and put things away till the next spring.

An old-timer told me about a farmer friend who decided quite early in the season that he had made all the syrup his family required, so feeling sorry for a neighbour who had no equipment, offered to let him use his set-up for the remainder of the season. This neighbour had never made syrup but was delighted to have a chance and proceeded to carry on vigorously. Time went on and one day the owner decided to go and see if his neighbour had picked up the buckets and other equipment, as he had promised to do when he had finished. "If you don't mind," he said "I would like to make it all summer."

There was another job for the men during this period, and that was to slaughter pigs in order to have meat for the summer. No fresh meat was sold at the store, but one farmer used to butcher quite often during the summer and peddle the meat throughout the community. That is the way we secured most of our fresh meat. The spring pork had to be canned or salted. Sometimes it was packed in brine in large crocks. Another way of keeping it was to slice and fry the meat, then pack it in layers in a crock. The fat that had cooked out of it would be poured over it while hot. If there was not enough fat, extra lard would be used to seal it. The meat would be weighed down with a large stone and would be dug out as required. A nice change from salt pork!

About the first thing the boys thought about in the spring was sucker fishing. In fact, both old and young took part in that sport. Along about the first of May some of the small swift streams would be practically alive with suckers, and the most exciting method of catching them in those days was by spearing them after dark. It really was great fun, but I found them too fast for me. Suckers do taste good if they are caught while the water is cold, and especially after a winter without fresh meat or fish. The only drawback is the bones which are so fine, so numerous and most elusive. I heard one boy remark, "I've been eating so many suckers lately, I can't get my shirt off!" By canning them, however, the bones soften and break up.

Spring is a wonderful time of the year in the country. Before the last patches of snow have disappeared, green shoots would poke up through the ground and the hillsides would take on a greenish tinge. One can almost see the buds opening up, and the treetops would suddenly turn from black to green. In no time the woods would be carpeted with wild flowers. Trilliums, which I had never seen before, grew in abundance along the roadsides. Large flocks of wild geese could be frequently heard and seen overhead on their way northward.

One afternoon in May, I called at Tory Hill School and was met at the door by the teacher, who smilingly said, "You may not want to stay long today." Before she could say more the children all laughed. I was wondering what this was all about, then the teacher told me the story. During the noon hour several of the children went into the woods and dug all the leeks they could find. They ate some themselves and brought the rest back for those who had stayed behind. The idea was that, definitely, the teacher would not be able to stand the aroma that would permiate the school, so would dismiss them for the afternoon. "But," she said, "I fooled them. I just ate some too!"

I had never heard of leeks and it was a few minutes before I caught the meaning, but I certainly noticed an obnoxious odor. When I told her I had no idea what leeks were, she asked the children if anyone had any more and practically every hand went up. She sent one boy to the cloakroom for some and he brought his lunch box, which was full of leeks. They looked to me like small green onions except that the leaves were flat rather than tubular. He offered me some, suggesting that I eat them then and there, but, remembering the call I intended to make on my way home, I said I wouldn't dare but would take a few home and try them later. It took a bit of courage to inspect the children that afternoon, especially their throats and teeth, but I managed.

Not many of the inhabitants made maple syrup, nor did the majority go sucker fishing, but one activity that involved every home was the spring housecleaning. Those were the days before Mr. Clean or Spick and Span, so many of the housewives relied on their own homemade soap to scour away the scars of winter, as well as using it for their laundry.

Soap making was another job that had to be done. Hardwood ashes were saved and put into a leach barrel (a large wooden barrel with a hole near the bottom) which was kept for that purpose. This was used to get the lye required in the soap making. Water was poured onto the ashes and, as it passed through them, it ran out the hole into a trough and on to a container. All fats were saved throughout the winter, especially from beef or venison. The fats were melted, then strained into a large iron kettle which was hung by tripod over a fire. To it was added the lye solution and, as the mixture heated, it was skimmed and skimmed until no more scum appeared, then poured into flat boxes. As it cooled, it was cut into the desired size cakes.

The first warm sunny day would be the signal for the housewives to begin housecleaning. And what a ritual that was! Most homes in town had two stoves. A cook stove in the kitchen and a box stove in the living room. Stovepipes usually ran through the ceilings and through rooms upstairs and finally into the chimney, giving off heat on the way. As soon as it was warm enough to do without the box stove, it was moved out to the woodshed, along with all the pipes

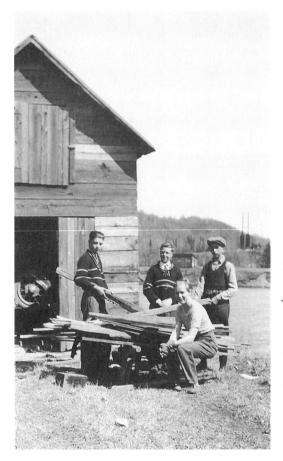

A work bee at the Outpost finds local boys (Murray Agnew, Ross Johnston and Jim Miller) helping house-keeper, Aileen Ames (seated) tidy up the back-yard. Note the head frame of the Graphite Mine in the distance. *Courtesy Wilberforce Heritage Guild Collection, donated by Aileen Ames Walker.*

which would be cleaned and stored away, then every room would be gone over thoroughly. Usually a new coat of paint was applied, or new wallpaper. Often two or three women would help each other at this job. It certainly wasn't considered a man's work!

The yards and lawns were next. It was surprising how dirty and untidy everything looked when the pure white blanket of snow had melted. The farmers too, cleared up their land, sometimes by means of burning a fallow (land that had previously been plowed and not seeded). In such cases they have to be very careful, as fire can very easily get out of hand.

This very thing happened one day shortly after I got my car. Smoke was sighted to the south and every available man, plus all the women there was room for in the cars, rushed to the scene. I took a load of women and followed to the home of George Barnes at South Wilber-

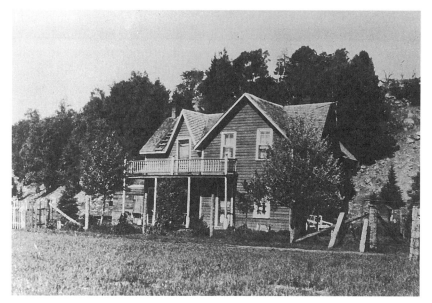

Pleasant Valley Farm, the home of Eva (Croft) and George Barnes, was located beside the site of the fire in the fields and woods, described by Gertrude LeRoy Miller. *Courtesy Wilberforce Heritage Guild Collection.*

force. There we learned that the fire had spread from a fallow that was being burned, and that it had got into the woods behind the Barnes home. The District Fire Rangers had arrived and were directing operations. Fortunately, the river was nearby and water was being carried to protect the house.

This house was a two-story building with a front porch and a balcony above. A large oak barrel stood on the ground under the eaves to catch rainwater and it was decided that, if that barrel were up on the balcony and filled with water, it could be used to great advantage in protecting the house. The problem was to get it up there. Someone ran to the barn for a ladder and Del (my hero) hoisted the barrel onto his shoulder, climbed the ladder and set it on the balcony floor. Afterwards he could never understand how he did it, but it goes to show the possibilities of latent strength emerging in a crisis.

We women didn't do much fire fighting, but realizing there were many men to be fed, set to work under Mrs. [Eva] Barnes' direction. I can just imagine what would happen if a group of about fifty hungry men should arrive unexpectedly at a city home on a day when all the stores were closed. They wouldn't fare nearly as well as these did at this farm home. Mrs. Barnes had been shipping eggs to the city, but there was a whole crate or more that wouldn't be going. A large baking of homemade bread was on hand, as well as rolls of homemade butter, pickles, maple syrup, preserves and food supplies. Towards evening the fire was brought under control and the men could come in, a few at a time, for rest and food. My job was to stand at the big cook stove and fry eggs. I never broke so many eggs in my life!

There was always a race in the spring to get a man with a team to prepare the garden plots in town. First he would come with a wagon and draw out and spread the manure that had accumulated at the stables during the winter. Next he would plow and harrow the soil. Before long the housewives would be raking and planting seeds. The children helped by planting the little onion sets and dropping potatoes in the prepared furrow. For the next few weeks the greeting would be, "Good morning. Got your garden all in yet?"

I arrived home quite late one night expecting to find the Outpost in darkness, but instead I found Aileen deeply engrossed in a seed catalogue! She smiled rather sheepishly as I walked over and peeked at what she had written on a sheet of paper. Not petunias or zinnias or asters, but carrots, beets, cucumbers, cabbage, and goodness knows what else, but all vegetables. When she saw my surprise she laughed. "You know," she said, "I believe I would like to have a garden. Have you any objections?"

I considered the matter for a minute or two before I answered. We had always a little garden at home but I'd had little to do with it, but I knew how nice it was to have fresh vegetables. It was always Dad's job first thing in spring, to spade up a patch in the backyard, usually about ten by fifteen feet or so. Well, I thought, possibly between the two of us we could spade up a little patch. (I didn't know then about quack grass).

"I think it would be a splendid idea," I said. "We could both work at it in our spare time. Yes, I think it would be fun."

"Well," said Aileen, "If you don't know anymore about gardening than I do, we both have a lot to learn!"

"I guess we can't learn any younger. Let me see that book."

So that matter was settled. But where should we start digging? The backyard was at least fifty feet by one hundred feet, with the driveway along the north side. We finally decided to wait until daylight to pick out a suitable spot, so we just concentrated on what to plant. Contemplating a lengthy session, Aileen thought we ought to be fortified with coffee, so leaving me to draw a few plans for us to work on, she slipped out to the kitchen. In a few minutes she returned with a plate of sandwiches and a pot of coffee. That really was a mistake, because the first thing we knew it was 2 a.m.! By that time we had spaded up a good sized piece of ground, planted potatoes, corn, onions, carrots, peas, cabbage, lettuce, radishes, and cucumbers. We had pulled a few weeds and watched the vegetables grow, and how we enjoyed eating them! In fact, we had given baskets of things away to our less ambitious friends!

I had planned to visit a school the next morning and would be leaving about 8:30 a.m. But I guess neither of us had ever really looked at that yard before. One look was enough to make us wonder what had ever made us think of a garden!

Last night we had forgotten about the pile of old lumber and junk that took up one large area. The furnace wood had been piled along the other side to dry, and bark and chips were scattered over the whole yard. And, to our horror, we realized that the lakeshore had evidently been used as a dump for years, where bottles, tin cans, and all kinds of debris had just been thrown over the bank. The ground had evidently not been cultivated for years, except for a little piece just behind the building. Well, we might be able to plant something in that strip.

I put all thoughts of gardening out of my mind for the day. However, that evening Del dropped in and we told him of our plans and enthusiasm of the night before, and how discouraged we were now. He just laughed, and said that there were great possibilities in that yard. We said that if there were, we would have to be shown, and if he would just go out and look at it he would feel the same as we did. He felt that it could be cleaned up and made into a good garden, and made some suggestions as to how to begin. Thus, we were in for another night session, but one that did not last as long.

The outcome was that Del promised to come over in his spare time and help clean up the yard. He would borrow a team and wagon and draw all the cans and junk to the dump, then he would saw up the old lumber to stove length and we could pile it neatly for burning as summer wood for cooking. A bonfire would take care of the rest. He suggested that instead of trying to spade up a small plot, we should hire someone to plow the whole yard and work it up well, get some fertilizer and plant a real worthwhile garden, as well as a nice patch of lawn. He thought that the lakeshore would be fine for cucumbers, not only because of the moisture, but the lake would protect them from early frosts.

Everything worked out well and we really did have a garden to be proud of, even though we had to hoe and pull weeds. We had lovely fresh vegetables all summer and when pickling time came we had so many cucumbers we gave them away by the basketful, just as we'd planned in the first place. When we didn't know what to do with all the cabbage, someone suggested that we make sauerkraut, so I purchased a six gallon earthenware churn and invited several friends in one evening to help shred cabbage.

To make sauerkraut, the cabbage is shredded very finely, packed into a crock, sprinkled with salt and pounded until the juice comes up. The pounder was usually made of a large chunk of hardwood on the end of a pole. More cabbage is added and the process continued until the crock is filled to within six inches or so of the top. It is then covered with cabbage leaves, followed by a large plate, and weighted down, usually with a big stone, so that the juice is forced to come up. The crock is then put in a warm place until it stops "working," usually about six weeks. If you can stand the odour of it until then, you will enjoy eating it. After it stops working it can then be placed in a cool place or even outside to freeze and used as needed. Or it can be sealed in jars.

While gardening was a novelty for Aileen and me, it was regular spring routine in other homes. Once the things started to grow, the children had plenty of work with the hoe to keep them out of mischief. And by the time school was out, wild strawberries were ready to be picked.

There was something fascinating about picking berries, but wild strawberry picking is a real backbreaking job, for they grow on small plants very close to the ground and are usually very small. I soon learned that if you do not pick them clean, that is, without the stems, you are a disgrace to the community. (I was used to buying tame ones.) Raspberries are different. Big juicy red berries hang under the high branches of the bushes just waiting to fall into your hand when you touch them. The temptation with raspberries is whether to transfer them from hand to your pail, or to your mouth! One mother solved that problem with her children by giving each a stick of gum when they started out. When they returned with their berries their gum would be put away until the next trip. I remember one woman was telling her neighbour about a wonderful patch she had found. She said she picked two twelve-quart pails and for every berry she put in her pail she had put two in her mouth!

At the end of the berry season the women compared notes. One would have 200 quarts altogether, another would have more, but it always had to be in the hundreds. And they really did! I could never quite figure out what they did with so many, but later, after enjoying meals in so many of their homes and tasting the delicious pies and preserves, and noticing the healthy appetites, I wondered no longer.

With all of these resources so readily available, the Depression at first did not affect this rural area so drastically as the cities. Wild game was in good supply, especially rabbits and partridge, also deer, if one didn't get caught killing them out of season. And it is surprising how good bear steaks taste! I helped eat several of that species. And there were lots of fish in the lakes. Fuel too was easily obtained. If they owned no woodlot of their own, villagers could obtain cutting rights from the government or private owners of woodlots. All that was required was the energy to cut the trees down, haul them home and cut and split them to suit their stoves. One could usually tell what sort of provider the man of the house was by the size of his woodpile. The proper method was to cut a year's supply ahead in order to have dry wood to burn, but some just cut it as required and their poor wives had the extra burden of trying to keep the home warm and do the cooking with green wood. If there was sickness in the home, the

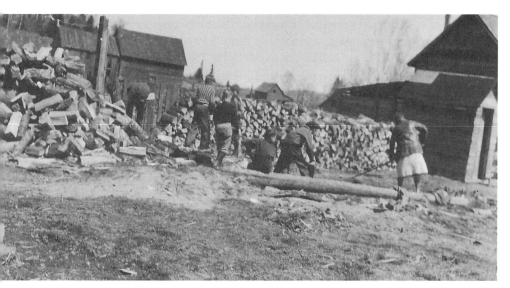

Many pitch in to help saw, split and pile the wood for winter, and to clean up the Outpost yard. Note the "biffy" to the left. *Courtesy Wilberforce Heritage Guild Collection, donated by Aileen Ames Walker.*

neighbours would have a bee and cut enough wood to see the family through the winter.

Our community was responsible for the upkeep of the Outpost, so in order to provide fuel[3] when funds were low, wood bees were organized. Usually someone who owned a large wood lot would offer all the wood that could be cut in one day, so the object was to get as many men as possible to give their time. Sometimes as many as twenty would turn up. Those with teams would draw the wood to the Outpost as poles and, during another day, these would be cut into proper lengths for stove and furnace by a buzz saw (a circular saw run by a gasoline motor). And yet another day, they would be split and piled to dry.

People were very good to help in this way, but one thing seemed very strange to me, though I suppose it is the same everywhere. Those who were most eager to help rarely needed the service of the Red Cross, while those who were always calling for assistance often were "too busy" or had some other excuse.

Another necessity at the Outpost was ice. The men cut large blocks when it was thick enough on the lake, drew it to the icehouse, and packed it in sawdust. It usually averaged about two feet in thickness and the supply would last most of the summer.

As time went on, the Depression struck harder and harder. The price of lumber dropped and wages in the mills dropped accordingly. In logging camps men were getting from $12 to $18 per month plus their board, if they could get a job. The Department of Northern Development decided to build some roads to open up this country, so camps were built and bus loads of men were brought up from Toronto to work on what is now Highway 35.[4] The machinery provided consisted of picks, shovels and wheelbarrows. Even the rock drilling was done by hand. Of course, many of the men had never handled these "complicated" machines before, nor had they ever been introduced to camp life, all for wages of fifteen cents an hour plus board. Other road jobs were created for local men. If they wanted to work, they had to send their names in and a certain number would be drawn every two weeks for two weeks work at a time. Each man was paid $1.20 per day (ten hours) and was charged 50 cents per day for board. If the men were lucky enough to live within walking distance (2 to 4 miles) of these jobs, which were in various parts of the county, it didn't cost them quite so much to live. Some boarded in private homes nearby, while some put up tents and boarded themselves, though it is hard to understand how they could live in tents at 30 to 40 degrees below zero. Sad to say, it did cost one local young lad his life. He died of pneumonia.

Some of the men turned to trapping, where they could work in their own time and as hard as they wished. And in spite of low prices for fur, they did quite well and working conditions were more pleasant.

Times continued to grow harder, but still most people tried to pay their own way. Nursing services were the same for everybody, whether they could pay or not, and those who made an effort to pay did not always do so in cash. Often it was a piece of fresh meat if they had killed a pig, a cow or chickens. It could be eggs, homemade butter, potatoes, whatever might be available.

Some of the teachers had great compassion for the children in their schools and spent a good portion of their meager salaries (about $650 per year) on food and clothing for them. One teacher in particular had a family near her school who really took advantage of her kindness and tender heart. There were seven school-age children in the family with at least two or three others who were too young to go. The mother would keep the school-age ones home because "they had nothing to wear." The teacher would buy each an outfit and they would attend regularly for a while, wearing the new clothes constantly, possibly night and day. Before long they had "nothing to wear" and would stay home until the teacher did something about it. This teacher helped the children plant a garden in the spring. During the winter she would secure a large soup bone and make soup for the children's lunch and, during the real cold weather, she would freeze the bone and use it again and again.

That was one advantage of our extremely cold weather, food was easily kept fresh. I often saw huge pieces of meat hung high on an outside wall of a building where no animal could reach it. It would be frozen solid and covered with ice. When they wanted a fresh roast they would get it down, saw off a piece and hang the remainder up again.

The Depression also halted the plans to open a Red Cross Outpost in Haliburton, a project which had been started in 1928. The people had progressed as far as to have received their Charter in August, 1930, and, to make matters worse, the Municipality of Dysart et al, which included Harcourt Township and Kennaway, went into bankruptcy. Neither were funds available to pay either the teacher or the school board.

Hazel [Miller, who was a teacher at Kennaway] found living conditions far below anything she had been used to, especially the food situation. She'd always had the best and plenty of it. Here there was little variety, mostly potatoes, beans and bread, with no butter or even any substitute. Sometimes the people were fortunate enough to have venison or fish. She had to carry her lunch to school which sometimes consisted of potato or boiled bean sandwiches. No wonder she was glad to get home whenever possible, and would take food back with her. Mrs. C. [a parent of some of her students] was a great help. She often snared rabbits and made stew for all the school children at noon. Toward the end of the winter the food situation became so bad that Hazel was almost ill. She told me about it in a letter that I passed on to her family. The next morning her father set out walking with a large pack on his back. This food she kept at the school, so she was able to eat well for awhile. She was not a bit sorry when that school term ended. Not many teachers had quite such difficult situations.

10

Recollections from a Watchful Neighbour

One day in 1971, I decided that it would be interesting to record some of the history of the early days in this community as told by one who was actually a part of it. So with my tape recorder, I visited an old friend and neighbour, Mrs. Isabel Graham Shay.

When I arrived at the Outpost, Mr. and Mrs. Bill Shay were our next-door neighbours. Bill was section man on the railroad and she kept a little variety store in the village. I was with Bill when he passed away during my stay there and, from then on, Mrs. Shay lived alone, except for her numerous cats which were a great comfort to her.

She seemed delighted when I told her of my plan to tape some of her memories and did not hesitate to talk when I asked a few questions. Mrs. Shay was born June 4, 1887 and her mother[1] died when she was quite young, leaving son Clark, and three daughters, Alice, Isabel and Ella. Her father, William Graham, and his recently widowed sister Mary Anne Clark, along with her daughter Bertha and sons Walter and Jack, raised both families together on their farm along the Haliburton Road, near the railroad where there was also a siding. Her story follows:

"It was like a hotel at our place. Everybody that came off the train came to our place. When they were loading logs or [railway] ties or

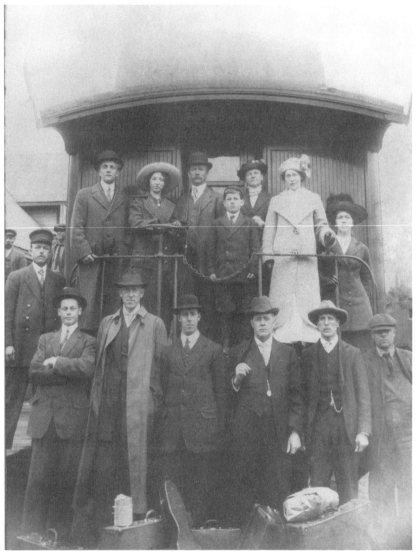

Isabel Graham (later Shay) was among this group of Wilberforce people who trav-elled to Bancroft to perform a play, circa 1913. From left to right (excluding three figures in the background), Back row: Herb Card, I.B.&O. conductor; Herb Schofield; Miss Addison; Mr. Addison; W. A. (Willie) Riley, the boy; Mrs. Addi-son; Isabel Graham; Bertha Clark. Front row: Reg Hamblyn; Mr. Smith; Reverend Percival Knight (Anglican Minister); _____, a railway supervisor; Frank Schofield; Frank Askey (with I.B.&O.). *Courtesy Wilberforce Heritage Guild Collection, donated by Nora M. Riley, wife of "Willie" in the picture.*

anything down on the siding, you see, the railroad ran right through my uncle's place; well, all these men were boarding at our place. So when all these men were all there, there would be about thirty of us, eleven of ourselves, counting my grandmother, aunts and children. We had good times at school too. You know where those big trees used to be by your church², only it was the old log church then down there. They were lovely trees at that time and they had a swing there. Before that they had a swing up back of the church, up on top of the hill. There were some big trees up there and someone had fixed a swing for us, a rope swing, and we used to go up there to swing before we got the other one down by the church. And there was a town hall. It was right between where the church is and Mrs. Croft's.³ The school used to be where Mrs. Croft's house is. The hall was built lengthwise, this way, and the church went the other way. They used to have fairs there every fall. Highland Grove, Gooderham and Wilberforce would all go together to put on these fairs, and they were pretty good. They used to bring their horses and oxen,…to show. Well, when there wasn't any fair there (here she had a spell of real hearty laughter), there were all these tables, benches and planks and things inside. We'd put planks across between the tables and run around there, you could hear us for a mile, chasing each other.

"The church was the old log church. There was never a foundation under it and later it was sagging so they tore it down and built the one that's there now. I can remember when they built it, I think I was about 16 or 17. The minister and all the men he could get were building it.

"There was a cheese factory right in front of where Bill Young's house is. Mr. [John] Dillman had a little store down there at the end of the bridge. It was quite a big place, the living quarters and a little long store at the front. Mr. [Lyman] Dillman used to have it. His people were pretty well to do out in Lindsay, and I guess they set Lyman up two or three times. It was hard to make things go. People didn't have much money in those days. If you did have a farm and could raise most of your own food it wasn't so bad, as there were no big stores up here until the railroad went through. Then a man by the name of Watson built one of these slant-roofed buildings, high at the front and slanted back. It was up where the railroad crossed the Burleigh.⁴ It wasn't a great big store. I was never in it. Then the railroad built their own store, the one that I used to work in for so many years. It was right along the railroad."

I asked her about her schooling.

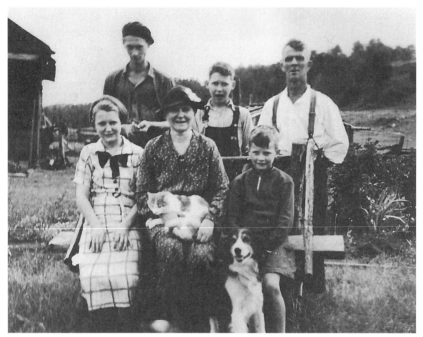

Wilfred Croft, a farmer and World War I veteran met the recently widowed May (Schofield) Barker, of England, on a train as she was emigrating to Canada to be with her Uncle Alfred Schofield. A major booster of the Red Cross, May Croft lived to be 103 years of age. She died in 1992. Wilfred Croft is in the back row, right; beside him is his son David; beside David is Herbert Barker, May's son born in England. In the front row (left to right) are Doreen Croft, May Croft and Mel Croft. *Courtesy Wilberforce Heritage Guild Collection.*

"I went to school till I was about fourteen. We went till we tried our entrance,[5] you see, then we went to High School in Minden.[6] My sister[7] and I went just one winter. You see, our father and mother were dead and we had to depend on our uncle to give us money as we had to pay our board and buy books. We went to school only three months, now the kids go, some of them till they're married, but we never got that chance. Then, after I quit going to High School, the Inspector gave me a school, he gave permits you see. I went away to South Monmouth. You remember where Mrs. [Florence] Perry used to live, well two or three miles beyond that. There was Hadlington and where they sent me was South Monmouth. You had to go through the bush part way and past Fred Perry's place. Fred was practically raised at our place from the time he came out from England as a kid. He was only ten when he came out with these Bernardo Boys.[8] He

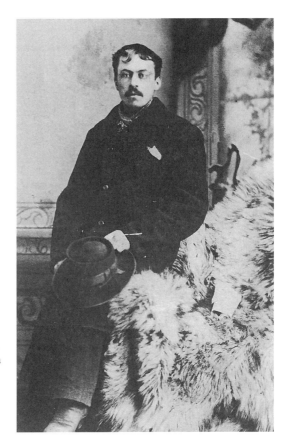

Lyman Dillman lived in South Wilberforce. His father, John, in addition to having 480 acres of land in the area, operated a store in this early settlement. Circa 1895. *Courtesy Wilberforce Heritage Guild*

practically grew up at our place. Our place was sort of a foster home. We also had Jim Mackness[9] whom we practically raised. And we had another boy for a while until he was old enough to go out on his own. Our folks were good-hearted that way and, of course, when they weren't going to school they could help a bit.

"I guess I was between 16 and 17 when I started to teach. The Inspector gave me a permit and I was just teaching a month when he gave Ella, my sister, a school at Hotspur. Jim Mackness was married and living there so she boarded at Jim's.

"I had about a quarter of a mile through the bush to walk to my school, but I didn't mind that, but there was a bear come out one night when Mr. Bolton was going through. I boarded with these people from Essex by the name of Bolton. There were a lot of squatters down there. People would come up and locate lots of timber. They didn't stay there themselves, so they would put squatters to look after their property

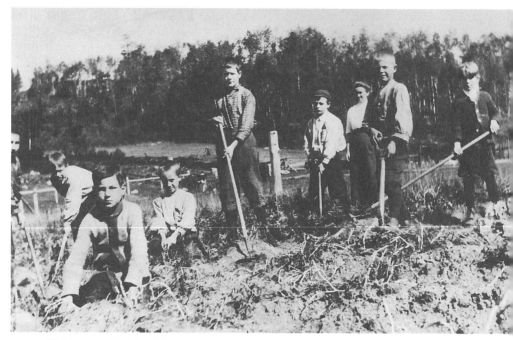

Children working in a Victory garden in the Wilberforce schoolyard. In the fore-ground left, kneeling on the ground is Bill "Willie" Riley; the boy with the hoe at the extreme left is Del Miller. *Courtesy Wilberforce Heritage Guild Collection.*

while they were away. Some of them were bachelors. Mr. and Mrs. Bolton were from Essex, but I don't know how they got away back there. They were a lovely couple and they had three little girls. I had about fifteen kids and they had never gone to school before. They built this lovely school down there but just like they built most of the schools, it was a rocky place and the yard wasn't really a good place for the children to play. Trees had been cut down and stumps left. They built this nice new school and they were just painting the door when I went down. Uncle Tom[10] took me down and over this road where they'd cut trees. The stumps would be so high and the road narrow, the wheels would strike the stumps and we had a real jolty ride from Fred Perry's[11] in to where I was to teach. I was there a month before I ever got home. I came out to Fred's and he and I walked out all the way from South Monmouth to my aunt's. We walked twelve miles to the party that was there that night.

"At school the children never had any religious training at all like we did, going to Sunday School and such, so I used to put verses from the Bible on the blackboard and they would memorize them. When the Inspector came he thought that was a good idea. I taught them to sing and things that the poor kids had never had the chance to do before. There was only one boy, 15, the Marshall boy, and away down four miles further on there were two fair size girls. They walked the four miles to school all the time I was there and never missed a day. I walked home with them one day. Their mother used to visit with the lady where I boarded. Mrs. Bolton's brother had married one of this lady's daughters. The mother was a friendly person. The girls wanted me to go home with them one night so I did. We walked out to school the next morning and were there at nine o'clock! I kind of enjoyed it, you know. Then the storekeeper, I don't know what he thought I was, he and his wife wanted to go away and he wanted me to look after his store, which was a couple of miles further, and me teaching all day! I had to refuse that, of course.

"I was there three months the first year, because they had just got the school built. Then I went back and was supposed to stay the year. Well, the Boltons were all right, but some of the others that lived down there were always fighting and I didn't like that. I quit three months before my year was up because the Boltons were moving up this way, up here by the bridge. Mr. Riley had a house up here, a log house, for them to live in. Mr. Bolton had worked for Mr. Riley a lot, and before that he used to come up here for groceries and carry them twelve miles home. So when the Boltons left, the only other place I could stay was Mr. Woods' or Mr. ? I can't think of his name, but he had a big family so all their beds would be taken up. His second wife was a girl from here at Highland Grove. I had known her before she was married to him. When he lost his first wife, they had some small children. I don't know how he came to meet this girl. I was down there one day for dinner. They wanted me to come down and they used me well, then I went down one evening when the minister asked me to go down with him. He told me he had stayed there one night and had to sleep with a bunch of kids, and he said when one wanted to turn over they would yell "flop!" (At this point another burst of real laughter).

"Then I taught at Wilberforce, the old school up here in Sections 6 and 8.[12] It was quite a big school, a lot of big children as well as smaller ones. I was just there to finish out the year. Then when holidays came I went to Toronto to see my sister and didn't come back for a while, and in the meantime they got another teacher. I had taught up at Beech Ridge[13] before that for three years, then I taught here. The next year

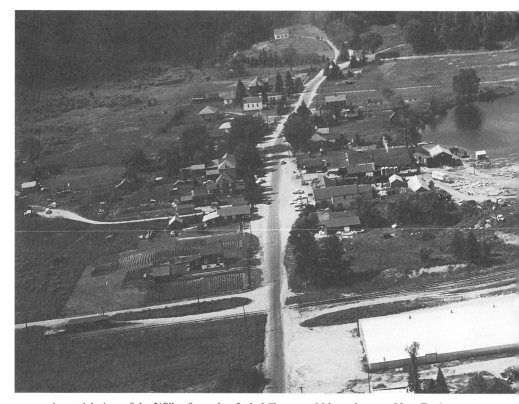

An aerial view of the Wilberforce that Isabel Shay would have known. Note Dark Lake with the veneer factory backing on to the lake. In the foreground, left, are Webber's gardens adjacent to the rail line and the railway station. The light roof is the Monmouth Arena. *Courtesy Wilberforce Heritage Guild Collection.*

they wanted me back at Beech Ridge, so I taught there for four years altogether. I boarded at Mrs. Mumford's, Bill Mumford's mother. She was a Pacey, Henry Pacey's sister, Alice. She was a good-natured woman, always laughing. There were thirty on the roll at Beech Ridge. They didn't have a school at Harcourt and they used to teach in a little wee shack and there were quite a number of children; so when they had a school meeting they decided to send the children over to my school, that's why I had so many. Later they built a new school in Harcourt. Ada Pacey[14] was one of my pupils, along with her sisters and Russell. There were two Scott girls and a little boy that died, a cute little fellow with brown eyes.

"I had a nervous breakdown so Dr. Walker told me to quit teaching. So I went to work in George Earle's[15] store. It was a very busy store. They used to come from Cheddar and all over. It was just like Agnew's store now, only it wasn't Red and White. People used to drive in with their wagons or buggies. In those days there were no cars, but they came from miles around. And the train came right through here. George made money here but not all from the store. He used to buy stuff from all along the line and ship it out. When he left here to go to Haliburton he was pretty well fixed, you know. Before he started up here he worked in camps and saved up his money, then he went to Belleville Business College. Hattie [Earle] was the youngest girl in the family. She married Bob Croft. They were only school kids and they used to ride around on horseback like Jesse James, you've read about Jesse James. They would just go for all they were worth. She was a good horsewoman, of course living on a farm down there, they had horses. They'd go away down to South Monmouth and all over on horseback, tearing around the roads like mad. Hattie was kind of pretty, she was dark, and had dark curls. Ethel Hughey,[16] Mable's[17] sister, they used to get into fights. Ethel had loose flowing hair and they'd get into fights and pull hair and they'd cry. The teacher would have to part them while the rest of us kids were almost in fits laughing."

"Have you always been fond of animals?" I asked.

"So you see all my cats! Well, a lot of these kittens came here in the winter. People want them in the summer and they don't want them in the winter, so they just drop them here. I'm very tender-hearted and can't see them starve. A lot of the big ones just came here, then the mothers had babies. It's surprising how many kids and women come in during the summer to see my kittens, so I've had great pleasure out of my cats. The kids seem to take quite a kick out of them. I was born to be very fond of animals.

"I never was afraid of anything when I was young. Ella, my sister, was very nervous and when we used to go to church at South Wilber-force at night, she'd clutch me tight coming past the Chemical Bush,[18] between Art Holmes' and the corner there. There were about a hundred Italians[19] cutting timber there. They had big camps down there and we used to meet these men; they were from 18 years to older men staying at camps. Of course, they would cook macaroni and other like food. They had their own way of cooking. They used to come to our place to buy a sheep or chickens for meat, and one day I was out feeding the chickens and a young fellow came and asked me, "Have you any checks?"

He meant chickens, you know, but I thought he meant a cheque

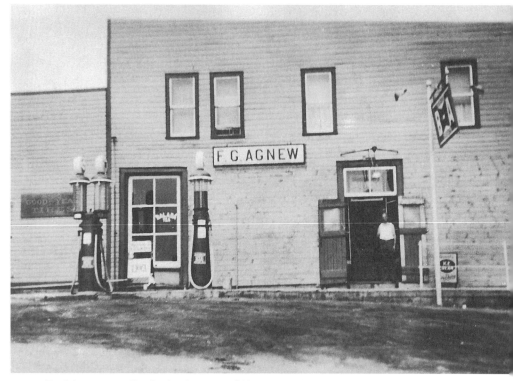

Fred Agnew standing in the doorway of his store in the early 1920s. Apparently it was unusual to see him without a shirt. Must have been a hot summer. *Courtesy Agnew Family Collection.*

and I said, "No, I have no cheque."

He said, "You lie! You have no check!"

"Well, when these men walked along the road they always walked in single file, and there was a hard path right down the centre of the road. They never walked along the side of the road and never walked two abreast like we do, but one behind the other. Ella and I would meet maybe eighty of them on our way home from school. At first we were a little nervous, them being foreigners. A lot of them couldn't speak English yet, but it was remarkable how quickly they picked it up. One year I had to stay home as Aunt Annie[20] was sick for three months in bed. Ally and Bertha[21] were in Toronto working, they were the two older girls, so I had to stay home for three months or more, and Ella said this young fellow went down to the school. He was a teacher in his own country, but he was only 18 and he wanted to learn our ways, and she said he learned so fast and was so comical.

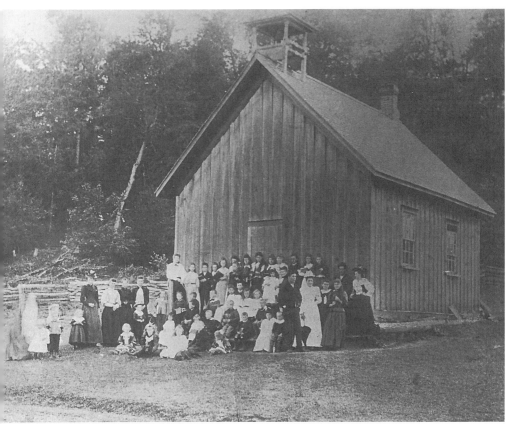

The first Wilberforce School, located in South Wilberforce (circa 1890s) was replaced in 1911 by the two-room Consolidated School, built several miles to the north. *Courtesy Wilberforce Heritage Guild Collection.*

"Maggie Ritchie[22] went to school too. She was forty years old, but she went to school to take penmanship and lower arithmetic because she kept the books for her father. He was one of the school trustees with my dad. We had more fun with Maggie over at that church. We used to go over to eat our lunch under the trees and she was really a scream. She used to keep us laughing our heads off. And Eva Croft,[23] with that bad foot she had! She was so lively and would go round and round the school about seven times hopping on one foot. A Hughey boy,[24] just a little fellow, called her "Heva!" "Heva!" he'd call, "If you don't stop that you'll hurt that dumb foot of yours!" We sure used to have fun at school. There were so many of us. We'd play ball and the teacher would come and play with us. One awfully hot day we were playing and she was running from one base to another and she fainted.

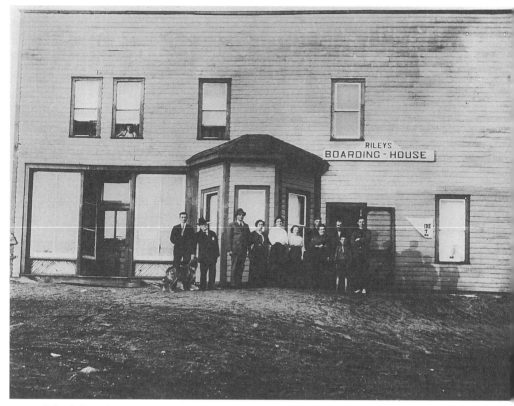

Riley's Boarding House, Store and Post Office was built in 1910 after the previous store and boarding house burned. The building picture here was purchased in 1919 by the Mulloys, who later sold to the Agnews. Located about 40 feet south of the present Agnew's store, the structure was destroyed by fire in the 1920s. The people (left to right) are: Hamlet Wolfraim, a student Methodist Minister; Dr. Neelands, a Lindsay dentist on his semi-annual visit to Wilberforce; Mr. Coville, Graphite Mine supervisor; Mary (Mame) Skuce; Letitia Skuce; Harriet Rowbotham, housekeeper; Ernest Riley; Martha (Mrs. Alec) Riley; Reg Hamblyn, boarder. Tom Sykes is looking out the top floor window. *Courtesy Wilberforce Heritage Guild Collection.*

I'll tell you, we kids doused lots of water on her! We brought her to in a hurry! We didn't spare any water! We had to carry our water from, well, you know where Don[25] has his house over there, well, we had to carry it either from there or Mr. Earle's. Mr. Earle[26] didn't like us getting water at his place, he was a very tight old man, and he'd tell us there were frogs and all kinds of things in the well so we wouldn't go there for water. There were so many kids, of course a pail of water wouldn't last long.

"I always think of my school days as very happy days because we had very good times. Ella said to me just before she died, "Bebe,[27] you always looked after me so good." Of course, she was a little younger. Coming across that lake down there one day, oh, was it ever cold! A cold wind, and she got to crying, she was so cold. We hadn't come very far from school,[28] just part way across the lake and she was pretty near frozen. I was just old enough to realize that if I tried to get her home without taking her in somewhere she really would freeze, so I took her into Mrs. Riley's. She had a good range fire on and we rubbed her. Mrs. Riley wanted us to stay all night. She was an odd old lady, you know, and sometimes she wouldn't speak and would be very grumpy. And other times she would be nice. Anyway, she wanted us to stay all night, but I was old enough to know that if we didn't come home they would be out looking for us, if we weren't there by a certain time. The lamps would be lit when we'd get home coming over the hills, so we could see our own house.

"One morning the snow was so deep when Ella and I started out, and we'd just got a little way from our farmyard when Uncle Tom called Ella back. He thought it was too stormy for her, but here I had to face it myself. Of course Ethel Holmes went to school, and Flossie[29] and Lylah,[30] one of the older girls for a while, and I'd join them at the next house. Then, when Blanche Stevenson got big enough to go to school, she went with us. If our boys or Uncle Tom were going to take the team and give us a ride, which they didn't do very often, we'd pick up these other kids and give them a ride too. I often think now the kids are drawn to school in buses and they don't know what hardships are. But there were no cars in those days, just horse and buggy or sleighs. We used to enjoy it because the horses would have strings of bells on and we'd sing those old songs.

"There was quite a lot of sickness. The doctor had to come from Haliburton, and Uncle Tom had to go for him, as there were no telephones. Many a hard trip Uncle Tom had for kids and everybody. Ella was three months old when our mother[31] died. The "grippe" is what they called it then. My mother and her brother and their mother, the three of them died in less than two weeks. Uncle Jim[32] went to my mother's funeral and was sick when he came home. He went to bed and was never able to leave it.

"Our folks were the only undertakers and they used to make the caskets. Aunt Annie and us girls used to cover them. They'd have them all lined with white inside, and they would make a pillow for the head. Aunt Annie had one of those crimpers to make lace to put around the edges. Later they'd have a breastplate on the top with the person's name and date of birth and death on it. If they wanted to make it extra fancy, they would have these fancy tacks that they tacked around, they would be in the shape of a star. They used to look pretty nice, you know."

11

No Routine Becomes Routine

A Red Cross Nurse in the pioneer years certainly enjoyed a life of diversity. I have been asked which branch of nursing I like best and find most interesting: maternity, schools, hospital nursing, bedside nursing in the homes…I really had no preference, but I believe I would find it very boring to have to stick to just one. I prefer a combination of all, which I found at the Outpost. I liked it because it took in the whole life cycle, not only of the family, but also of the community. Every phase of the work was most enjoyable.

By meeting the children at school, I was given a reason for visiting the homes and thus became involved with every age group. That was the nursing part, doing the work for which I had been trained. Some of the most thrilling parts were just getting there. Everything depended on communication (or lack of it), road conditions and weather; a trip to a patient so often involved many people besides myself. I have mentioned travelling the narrow crooked roads among the hills and through the bush by car. Some of those were exciting indeed to a newcomer.

Travelling during the winter was really exhilarating, especially for a city person. The heavy open sleigh with its deep layer of straw was a very comfortable way to travel in cold weather, but not too thrilling because the heavy workhorses always took their time. However, these same sleighs did provide some exceptional trips when dozens of people would pile on some evenings and drive to a farmhouse four or five miles away, over hills and through the woods, singing all the way. We always chose a bright moonlit night, but it did not really matter about the temperature as we were packed in quite tight. We could always get off and and walk for a while if we got cold. When we arrived at the farmhouse (Wilfred Croft's[1] was the favourite destination), we would play games, dance, sing, eat and have a wonderful time. Until someone would remind us that it was going to take us just as long to return to town, so we should be on our way. Strange to say, the return trip was always much quieter.

By far the snappiest way of winter travel was by horse and cutter, especially if the horse was one that could really step along. The music of the sleigh bells would delight anyone. I shall never forget the queer feeling I had in my stomach the first time I was driven by horse and cutter across a frozen lake. (Cutting across lakes and through fields and woods saved miles of travel during the winter). The hollow sound of the horse's hooves striking the ice really frightened me for I could not believe that the ice would be strong enough to support much weight. I had yet to hear about the log hauls when large sleighs, piled high with logs, were drawn across lakes to the lumber mills.

People from the city were always looking for excitement or thrills of one kind or another, and seemed to think that country folks led very dull lives. I would like to take them for a few trips like those I had on the gas-powered handcar, especially in the middle of the night, speeding through the darkness, hoping there was nothing on the tracks. Even a skunk or a porcupine could knock us off into eternity! This was by far the fastest means of travel in winter, but unfortunately the railroad tracks didn't run to every home so I often had a long walk at the end, unless I was met with another vehicle. Sometimes my calls coincided with the train schedule, but that did not happen very often.

The school van often provided a way for me to get to or from a patient. It carried children from the South Wilberforce area, some having to come five or more miles. At that time it was driven by Wilfred Croft. The winter van was a large box-like affair on runners, drawn by a team of horses. It had a door at each end, each with a small window that let in very little light. The front door had two little holes for the reins to pass through to the driver. A bench extended along each side and a small makeshift stove stood in the centre with the pipe protruding through the roof. Many a ride I had in that van and how sorry I felt for the poor children, about twenty of them, who had to spend

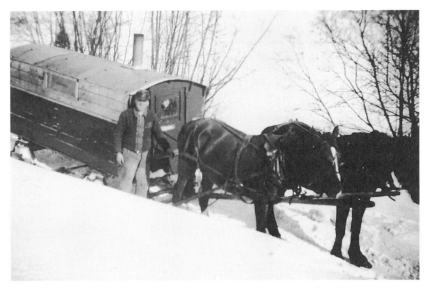

The school van, an enclosed vehicle, provided reasonably comfortable transportation for students in the winter. The driver here is believed to be Edward "Eddy" Earle. *Courtesy Ken and Nadeen Sanderson Collection.*

hours in it every school day during the winter. Some had to leave home long before daylight and it would be dark again when they returned after school. Often their lunches would be frozen by the time they arrived in the morning, for the thermometer frequently dipped to thirty or more degrees below zero. I am sure the children did not find these trips very thrilling! The summer van was the same type of outfit, only it was on wheels and open at the sides, with curtains to roll down in case of rain.

When the snow was almost gone and the frost coming out of the ground, I was to learn that it was the time to stay at home unless travel was absolutely necessary. Of course, the stork didn't realize that, and often sickness struck regardless of road conditions. Mud was the order of the day and the horses really earned their oats, but the nurse had to be ready for everything. Often I travelled by horse and buggy and, when the roads were really bad, a team and light wagon were the best means of getting around. I was always sure of transportation of one kind or another, and I found that having such a variety of ways was not nearly as monotonous as having to ride day after day on crowded streetcars.

Those were a few of the ways I had of reaching the sick. Sometimes I went by train and returned by handcar, but the most satisfactory way,

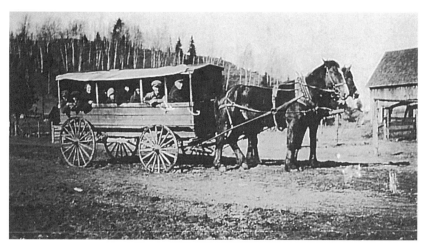

The summer van, also pulled by a team of horses, is shown here taking students home from school. It is likely that, Marjorie (Cronsberry) Pollock, the teacher of the Junior Room at Wilberforce School from September 1925 to June 1927, took the picture. Wilfred Croft is the man second from the right. *Courtesy Wilberforce Heritage Guild Collection, donated by Aileen (Young) Broughton (originally from Marjorie Pollock).*

of course with roads permitting, was by driving my own car. I became very brave about driving, even in bad weather. As those were the days before snow tires, I relied on chains, which fitted over the back wheels. They were used as much for mud as snow and, when the snow got too deep, the car was put away. Icy conditions were about the worst problem, especially on the hills. Whenever possible, I would take someone with me, as a little extra weight seemed to help, sometimes even when a person was standing on the back bumper. And a box of sand to sprinkle in the tracks was always carried!

Patients came to the Outpost by various conveyances too, but there was one that capped them all, which took place after I left and another nurse was in charge. The patient lived about half a mile away and, when labour began in the night, her husband did not want to leave her alone while he went to get the nurse to come for her. This was a real problem. He had no car, but he did have a wheelbarrow. Fortunately, his wife was a very small person and, by using a quilt for padding, it proved a very satisfactory conveyance.

I used to feel sorry for the doctors who had to travel such distances. When they could drive their cars it wasn't too bad, but at other times the trip was dreadful. So much time had to be spent on the road. They used to tell me to call them only if it was absolutely necessary, especially during the winter and spring months. I often received instructions by relayed telephone messages, and in that way many long hard trips were avoided.

Early one very cold morning I was on my way down to breakfast and happened to look out the front window in time to see a horse and cutter stopping at our gate. The driver looked half frozen with his fur collar and cap covered with frost. The horse was also covered with frost. It wasn't until he got out of the cutter that I recognized Dr. Frain from Haliburton! What could he be doing here at this hour? When I opened the door he seemed awfully surprised to see me. He said he thought I would be in Harcourt, seven miles further on. He had presumed that it was I who had sent the message, and he had set out at 4:30 that morning.

I tried to persuade him to come in and have some break-

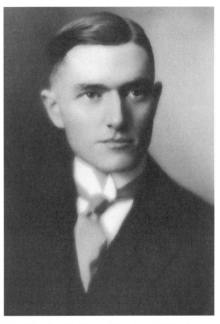

Dr. Charles E. Frain (October 1893–August 14, 1934) was a graduate from the University of Toronto in 1916. He served overseas in the Canadian Army Medical Corps during World War I. After taking more training and practising briefly in Toronto, went to Minden about 1920 and on to Haliburton in May, 1925. The rest of his life was spent in Haliburton. *Courtesy Dr. J. Bruce Frain of Winnipeg, Manitoba, son of Dr. Charles E. Frain.*

fast and get warm, but he was afraid the case was urgent and would not take the time. About noon he returned, and was he ever furious! He said it was a confinement, a first baby, and the husband had become very excited when his wife's pains began. He had rushed to the store, where the only telephone in Harcourt was located, and called Dr. Lumb at Bancroft, who was their nearest doctor who could have come by gas car in a few minutes. When he was told that Dr. Lumb was out on a case, the husband sent a message through to Dr. Frain, not realizing that it would take him several hours to make the trip. When Dr. Frain had not arrived by the time the husband thought he should, he tried once more to reach Dr. Lumb and succeeded. Shortly after Dr. Frain arrived, Dr. Lumb also appeared!

The patient was all right, Dr. Frain said, but would not have her baby for at least another hour or two, so he turned the case over to the other doctor and left. But first, he said he gave the husband a piece of his mind for not having called me in the first place, and I'd have known when to send for a doctor. Poor Dr. Frain! We gave him a good dinner before he started out on his homeward journey. I felt sorry for his horse too, but he said it had been fed at Harcourt. He said it belonged to Walter Payne, who lived about halfway to Haliburton, where he had left his horse that morning, so it would be fresh and ready to take him from there.

Many of my calls were to cases other than confinements. A message came late one afternoon after a big snowstorm. A woman at Beech Ridge was very ill and if I wanted to go to Harcourt on the train, which was due soon, I would be met there and taken to her home, (which was about three miles back toward Wilberforce). When I arrived I found Eddie Mumford,[2] a twelve-year-old boy, waiting with horse and cutter. By that time it was dark and 15 or 20 degrees below zero. How a horse can keep to the road in the dark, especially when it is drifted with fresh snow, is more than I have been able to understand. We just about upset several times as the drifts were very high and, with it being nighttime we could not be prepared for them. Of course the snow is nice and soft, and, as long as the horse does not get frightened and run away, a little upset hurts no one. But this time I was hoping we could make the trip without a spill, and we did.

At last we arrived at the log house at the top of a hill, across the road from my very first outpost patient. Mr. F. welcomed me and said his wife was upstairs and that a neighbour was with her. The downstairs was one big room. Since there was a good fire in the cookstove, I removed my wraps and warmed my hands before climbing the steep narrow steps. The second floor, like the first, was also one big room and it contained three double beds and a box stove that was throwing out tremendous heat. In the bed nearest the stove lay the patient, a woman who must have weighed at least 220 pounds, fully dressed and appearing very ill.

As a student nurse, one thing above all else was impressed on me: nurses never, no *never*, diagnose. The physician diagnoses the case and prescribes the treatment; the nurse carries out that treatment to the best of her ability. Well, here I was with a very sick patient and no doctor to diagnose and give orders. The best I could do was to examine her and use my own judgement regarding treatment. I found her temperature extremely high, but blamed the nearby stove as a partial cause. Her pulse was very rapid and her breathing fast and laboured. She coughed frequently and complained of pain in her chest. I pictured in my mind a row of beds on Ward 'B' facing open windows, with pneumonia patients in half sitting positions, and separated from the rest of the ward by screens to insure tranquility.

First of all, the patient's clothing had to be removed. This was accomplished with the help of the neighbour before she left with my travelling companion. She promised to return the next forenoon.

Pneumonia in those days before the advent of the wonder drugs, the sulfas and penicillin, was one of the diseases in which nursing was about the most important factor. The disease just had to "run its course." It is an acute infection of the lungs and the most fatal of all acute diseases, involving not only the lungs, but also the action of the heart and the whole circulatory and nervous systems.

In nursing a pneumonia patient, one had to prevent the patient from placing any unnecessary strain on the heart. Complete rest and quiet were essential, along with relief of the lung congestion, usually accomplished by the application of mustard plasters. As well, and it was necessary to turn the patient frequently and ensure lots of fluids and care of the mouth.

I gave this patient a warm sponge bath, which I repeated during the night and again in the morning, for the purpose of reducing her temperature and eliminating waste materials. I applied mustard plasters followed by warm camphorated oil at regular intervals during the night, gave her a few doses of cough mixture and persuaded her to drink a considerable amount of fluids.

By daylight my patient was sleeping quietly and her temperature was gradually approaching normal. When she finally awoke, she said she felt like a new person, and was ready for a light breakfast.

Evidently Mrs. F.'s illness had not developed into a real case of pneumonia and had been treated in time to prevent that, for her temperature stayed down, her pulse was steady and strong and her flesh was warm and dry. After breakfast I felt it would be safe to leave. I wrote down instructions regarding her care for her husband and neighbour, then began preparing for my walk to Wilberforce, as I knew of no other way to get there. I was just ready to leave when my companion of the night before stopped in, he said, on his way to town. This time he had his dog sled and offered me a ride, which I accepted very gratefully. Of course we could not ride at the same time, as there was only one big collie to pull, but whenever I got off to get warm, he walked along with me. I was very thankful not to have to carry my bag. That was my first ride on a dog sled and a very enjoyable one.

For the nurse to face a blizzard on a cold winter night in order to get to a patient was one thing, but for a woman who was in labour with her eighth child, to strike out under the same weather conditions to get to the nurse, was another matter entirely. About 2 a.m. on a February morning during a terrible blizzard, I was awakened by a loud pounding on the front door, as well as the ringing of the doorbell. "This must be urgent," I thought. Throwing my dressing gown around me, I hurried down the stairs with my flashlight. I opened the door and there stood Mrs. [Annie] Mumford, Eddie's mother, and her husband Arthur, both covered with snow and looking half frozen. I didn't have to be told she was in labour. As quickly as I could, I got her into bed. Aileen came down and, with hot water bottles and a hot drink, we soon had her warmed up. By the time Art had found a stable for his horses and returned, I had dressed and was ready for work.

She told us that they had been hours on the way. The storm was so bad that even the horses had lost their way and for some time they had no idea where they were. All the time she was having pains and was so afraid her baby would be born before they reached the Outpost. Fortunately, they had made it and about an hour later the baby boy arrived safe and sound. I hated to think what might have happened if they had not found the road when they did.

One way in which my work at the Outpost differed from working in a large hospital was that there was no regular routine to be followed. I always had to be prepared for anything that turned up. I was apt to be called at any hour, day or night in any kind of weather, either to go out or to attend someone being brought in. It might be a maternity case, a minor injury which I could treat myself, or a more serious one when I would merely administer first aid until the doctor's arrival. One man had walked six miles to see me about his rheumatism. He said he'd heard I was "real good on rheumatism." I gave him a bottle of wintergreen liniment, which I was sure would give him some relief. I never knew what was coming next, but one thing I could always be sure of was a call of one kind or another if I had made plans to attend a party, dance, or even a conference away from town. It seldom failed. Most often, of course, it was the stork, for it certainly had it in for me! Well, at least life sure was not boring!

But, of course, that was the purpose of my being here and I soon learned not to be disappointed when such things happened. Finally, I found it best not to make any plans, but to take things as they came. It was the safest way and it seemed more or less like opening the mysterious parcels under the Christmas tree, each a surprise complete in itself. And if I should happen to be extremely tired when something turned up, a rush call or an unexpected patient, I always seemed to receive an extra 'shot' of pep and would completely forget about my weariness.

One evening I received a message from Dr. Frain asking me to go to a certain home about eight miles away as soon as possible. That was the complete message so I did not know what to expect, but found the house packed with people. A young man was lying on the bed, apparently asleep, and the doctor was using his stethoscope on his chest.

When he saw me, Dr. Frain explained that this chap had been taking convulsions and that his condition was very poor. He had been with him for several hours and had received an urgent call from his office and had to leave. He would like me to stay and continue the hypodermic injections he had been giving the fellow. And above all, I was to try to get him to drink some water. So far Dr. Frain had been unsuccessful in doing that. The doctor asked me to report to him about seven o'clock in the morning, if the man was still living.

So I took over and Dr. Frain left, but none of the audience did! I had noticed that on various occasions that when anyone in that particular community was ill, all the neighbours seemed to swarm in. Whether it was to try to help or from curiosity, I never did figure out. In this case, though, I was quite sure that it was curiosity that brought the majority, for they had heard that this patient was taking "fits," and all wanted to see what they were like.

As soon as the doctor left, I looked around the room and counted eight people. Then, with the excuse of wanting to wash my hands, I walked through another room into the kitchen, counting the people as I went. There were 27 more! Thirty-five people in all! Speaking as kindly as I could, I told them that now that the doctor had gone, I thought the patient would rest much better if there were not so many around, so would they all please leave. They did so, very reluctantly. Soon all had gone, leaving only his mother and brother. I suggested that they go upstairs and try to get some rest, and if I should need them I would call. So, in a short time I had the place all to myself. What a relief!

Besides the hypos at regular intervals, I gave the patient a warm sponge bath, but he did not even rouse. His pulse seemed to improve, as did his breathing, but try as I would, I could not get him to swallow a drop of water. Around 2 a.m. he became a little restless, but I was still unsuccessful in that respect. Then, suddenly, about three o'clock he opened his eyes and started to get out of bed. I talked to him quietly and tried to prevent him from getting up. But he paid no attention, then said he wanted a drink of water! When I offered him what was there, he would not touch it. He said he wanted fresh water. His brother heard him and came down and brought water from the kitchen, but that wouldn't do. "No," he said, "I want fresh water and I'll go out and pump it myself."

I tried to get him back into bed while his brother dashed out to the pump, but he lashed out with his fist and broke the crystal on my watch. "Well," I thought, "If you are that strong you can just go out to the kitchen," so out he walked, in his shirt-tail! By then a pail of fresh water was on the table and he grabbed the dipper and proceeded to pour it into himself! We didn't think he was ever going to stop! Finally he said, "That's better," and walked back to his room, got into bed and in a moment was sound asleep!

On my way home shortly after 7 a.m., I stopped in town and called Dr. Frain as I had promised. Needless to say, he was mighty pleased with my report. We found out later that the illness had been caused by some moonshine the chap had been drinking.[3] He was soon completely recovered.

12

As Nurse's Role Expands, Families Do Too

The original purpose of having a nurse in Wilberforce, I was told, was mainly to care for mothers and infants at time of birth. It seemed to me that this purpose was being fulfilled to some extent, but I shuddered when I learned that there had never been a pre-natal program of any kind introduced. Those were the days when women did not tell anyone that they were pregnant until they couldn't keep the secret any longer. And even then it wasn't a subject to be talked about. I heard of one woman, a mother of nine, who told her husband late one night that he had better go for their neighbour right away. "What do you want with her at this time of night?" he asked.

"I'm having a baby and the pains have begun," was the reply. He didn't even know she was pregnant!

During my training I had seen more than one patient in convulsions, which often would be fatal. The Public Health aspect was the prevention of these, and many other conditions and complications, by recommending regular urine tests for albumin and general pre-natal check-ups, along with advice regarding diet, and exercise.

In the 1930s, the Department of National Health and Welfare put out booklets on pre-natal care on a monthly basis. Each dealt with one particular month of pregnancy, advising regular diet, precautions and general care. Whenever I learned of a woman in my area that was pregnant, I sent her name in and she would receive a booklet each month, the last dealing with baby care. I found these a great help in getting the women to realize the importance of pre-natal care. They also paved the way for any other health teaching I could give. I tried to impress on them the importance of having a doctor, but when they refused to call one and would send only for me, usually at the last moment, I just had to do the best I could, praying that everything would be all right.

Those were the days before the "pill" and Family Planning Clinics. Contraceptives were very "hush hush", but women told me about certain methods they had heard of and asked for advice. Nurses at that time were not trained in that respect, so my advice was for them to consult their doctor.

Consequently, large families were very common. Some poor women were practically worn out from having a baby almost every year. During the four years I was in charge, I attended some women three times. The largest family in my territory had been increased by two (a pair of twins) shortly before my arrival, which brought the number of the 79-year-old man's offspring to twenty-six. While I had seen six of his children at school, but knew nothing of the family background until the Welfare Officer came to see me about them one day, and enlightened me. This man, he said, had survived two wives and his present wife, who was the mother of his last twelve children, also was his eldest son's sister-in-law. With a bit of figuring, we decided that made that old fellow his son's brother-in-law and his grandchildren's uncle.

We were very proud of the work we were able to accomplish at our Outpost and the care we could give to our patients, but when women began coming from the city to have their babies, we thought we really must have something! The second winter I was in charge, a local woman[1] who had gone to the city and married, came home to have her baby at the Outpost. It was Sunday when she came to the door, and there was no way to get in touch with the doctor by telephone since all stations were closed. Someone had to be sent for him, a half-day's journey there and back. Fortunately, as this was her first baby, he managed to get there in time. Soon she had a lovely little daughter to take back to the city. About eighteen months later she returned to have her second daughter. In the meantime, yet another local woman returned to Wilberforce to give birth to her second child. She told me that she had made all the arrangements to have her first one in her home in the city, as the majority of women did in those days. She had

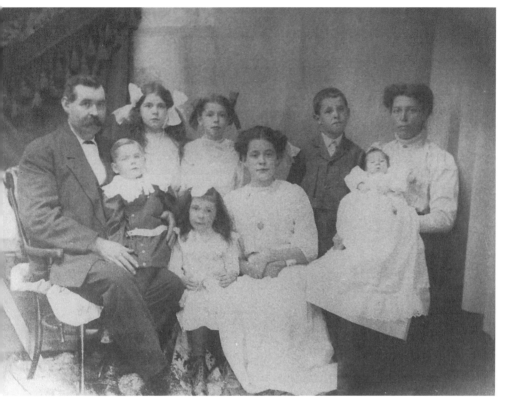

In the early 1900s, John and Minah Holmes came to Monmouth Township with their family. John purchased Lot 34, Concession 16 on which the present hamlet of Wilberforce is built. The photograph shows John and Minah with their children: Ruby; Daisy; Leonard; Johnny; Minah; Mildred and Leslie. *Courtesy Wilberforce Heritage Guild Collection*

arranged for both a nurse and a doctor. When labour began a few days earlier than expected, she could get neither a doctor nor nurse in time and had to deliver herself! What an awful experience for a woman who was having her first baby! So here she was at our little Outpost, 25 miles from the nearest doctor! We were able to get a message through to Dr. Speck and he arrived from Haliburton in the nick of time. This time she had both doctor and nurse.

About the busiest eighteen hours of my career took place in June during my third summer in Wilberforce. Early in the evening a patient was brought in by her husband. She was having regular pains, though her baby was not due for at least two more months. This was her first pregnancy. Her husband dashed down to the store and sent a message to Dr. Frain, who came as quickly as he could and in time to deliver the infant. But in spite of all our efforts to save her, the wee baby lived only about two hours.

It was well after midnight when Dr. Frain left, and I had just nicely got everything cleared away and was thinking of having a rest when another unexpected patient arrived. This time Dr. Speck was sent for and, after a very difficult delivery, this baby finally arrived just after daybreak, safe and sound.

I had arranged to hold a Baby Clinic at the Outpost that morning (not expecting to have any patients) and to give toxoid to the children at Wilberforce and Essonville Schools. Dr. Speck had planned to be at them all, but of course neither of us had figured on the stork's visit as well. He decided to stay and help with the clinic, so while I set everything up, the doctor had a rest. By 9 a.m. the mothers began to arrive with their babies and pre-school children. Several had come in the school van. I weighed and Dr. Speck inoculated twenty-seven infants and pre-schoolers, besides counselling the mothers on various matters. As soon as we finished there, we went across to the Wilberforce School where several doses of toxoid were administered and ten children were vaccinated against smallpox. Since there were several children waiting at Essonville School for their first dose of toxoid, Dr. Speck said he would stop in there on his way home and give it. I am sure he must have been as tired as I was when he finally reached home. I was certainly ready for a rest, but of course I had two mothers and a baby to attend to first.

I wondered sometimes how tired I would have to be in order to, with a clear conscience, refuse to go on a call. I never did get to that stage, for an extra "shot" of energy always seemed to come when needed. There was, however, one day when I was exceptionally tired. It was about the warmest June day that we'd had and I left the Outpost about 8 a.m. to give toxoid at the two Highland Grove schools, about 12 and 17 miles away. The children had all received their first doses so were not as nervous as they had been on my previous visit. Even so, it was a trying ordeal as two of the girls fainted, which of course upset the others. A few of the mothers brought their pre-school children for their toxoid, but some were unable to come so I went to their homes after finishing at the school. One family insisted that I stay for lunch and I was very glad to accept the invitation.

After lunch I proceeded to the next school and went through the same routine and, by about four o'clock, was ready to tackle the hills

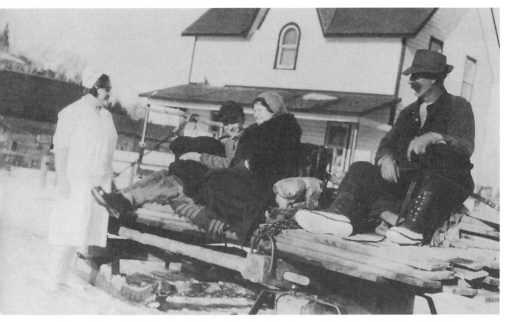

Nurse Gertrude LeRoy bids farewell to family of new baby, Joan McIntyre, held by father, Ken McIntyre, seated beside mother, Mabel McIntyre. Grandfather, Fred Barnes, with the reins, is about to take them home by horse and sleigh. *Courtesy Wilberforce Heritage Guild Collection, donated by Mabel (Barnes) McIntyre.*

on my homeward journey. In all, I had given 78 doses of toxoid and had visited ten homes.

Incidently, one must remember that those were the days before disposable needles and syringes. As I had very few of each to work with, each one had to be cleaned and sterilized many times. A portable little gadget that would hold a small pan of water heated by an alcohol lamp was always carried with my equipment.

At last I arrived home and decided that a nice cup of hot tea and a rest before dinner would make me feel much better. If only we had a shower, or even a bathtub! Well, I was just pouring my tea when the doorbell rang. It was Mr. W., practically out of breath. His son, Pat, had cut his foot with an axe and was bleeding very badly. Would I please come at once? He had come on horseback, so I assured him I would start at once. Hurriedly I gathered the things I might need and, forgetting all about my tea, off I went.

Fortunately, Pat's injury was not as serious as I'd feared, and it was soon fixed up and dressed. Of course, I was not permitted to leave without first having supper with them. Poor Aileen! She never knew

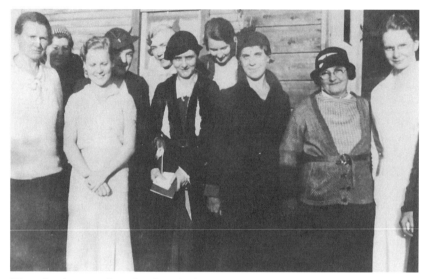

These local women have just heard a lecture on nutrition given by Red Cross dietition, circa early 1930s. They are: (from left to right) May Croft; Florence Perry; Aileen Ames; Gertrude LeRoy R.N.; Flora Marshall; Clara Schofield; _____; Eva Barnes; Sophia Sanderson and Miss Thompson, the dietition. *Courtesy Wilberforce Heritage Guild Collection, donated by Aileen Ames Walker.*

when I would be home for a meal.

After supper I decided to make some calls while I was in that neighbourhood and thus save making another trip, so it was after eight o'clock when I finally returned to Wilberforce. Strange to say, I was not nearly as tired as I had been when I poured that cup of tea. In fact, I walked up to the schoolyard and watched a ball game.

It was about ten-thirty when I arrived home from a confinement on another occasion. I was too tired to even open the gate to drive to the garage, and was about to leave the car there when Aileen came out to tell me about a message that had come for me. Mrs. H. had been kicked by a cow while milking, and was hurt quite badly. The family had been unable to reach a doctor. Naturally, I gathered up the necessary articles, and taking Aileen with me for company, left at once. We found the patient in terrible pain with a fractured leg. I was glad to be able to give her first aid and relieve her suffering until the doctor was available.

There were at least a few cases, I felt, that justified my being at the Outpost at that time. In each instance I was able to help save a patient from a great deal of suffering and possibly death. There was one woman who had not been well for some time. The roads were so bad, and having no way of getting to a doctor without a great effort, she just doctored herself with various remedies she'd heard about. Finally, one day she came to me for advice. I'd had considerable experience with diabetes during my training (insulin had recently been developed) and some of the symptoms she mentioned sounded very suspicious, so I had her bring me a sample of urine which I tested. Sure enough, I found a very strong sugar reaction. Immediately I arranged for her to see a Diabetes Specialist in Toronto, who soon had her under treatment.

A young couple brought their three-week-old baby to me to see if I could recommend a formula for him. The mother had been breast-feeding him, but lately he had been vomiting after every feeding and had also lost weight. I asked several questions and learned that he was quite constipated and that when he vomitted, it seemed to shoot out of his mouth.

Immediately, I remembered one of our university lectures on pyloric stenosis. Some of the symptoms were projectile vomitting, constipation, loss of weight and visible gastric peristalsis. Since the surgeon was to operate on such a patient that afternoon, he had brought the infant to the classroom so we could see for ourselves. With gastric peristalsis, a small "lump" seems to move across the stomach area. The muscle surrounding the entrance to the stomach will not permit the food to enter the stomach. When the food reaches it, the muscle tightens like a drawstring and shoots the food back.

I opened the baby's clothing and watched his little stomach, and there it was! So I explained it all to the parents and advised them to waste no time in taking him to Sick Children's Hospital in Toronto. If I had not known about pyloric stenosis, I would no doubt have kept trying various formulas until he would have eventually died of malnutrition. As it was, he had his operation and in a short time was as normal as any other child.

I had two maternity cases in which I suspected placentia previa and thus was able to do something for the women. This condition is the result of the placenta, or afterbirth, having developed partially or completely over the birth canal rather than in the upper part of the uterus. It loosens when dilation begins, thus causing a hemorrhage and sometimes preventing natural childbirth. My first such case was a mother of nine. She and her husband arrived at the Outpost by team and sleigh, one cold night in February. I hadn't even heard of the woman before, but of course that was not unusual.

After a fifteen-mile drive, which had taken about two hours, I wasn't surprised to find her very cold and tired. As we had a patient downstairs, Aileen and I helped her upstairs and into a nice warm bed while her husband set out to find a stable for his horses. She'd had all her other children at home with a neighbour in attendance, and she had planned to do the same this time, but with all the bleeding she thought there must be something wrong. "Trouble ahead," I said to myself, and to her, "I guess we had better send for a doctor right away."

"Oh, no," she said, "I didn't intend to have a doctor. I've always got along all right before."[2]

Well, I thought to myself, you may not want one, but you are having one just the same.

"I'll see what your husband says about it," I said.

As soon as he returned, I told him what I suspected and what might happen. I explained that if a doctor could come and bring special instruments, no doubt his wife could have a safe delivery. He immediately agreed and hurried to the store to see if he could get a message through to Haliburton or Bancroft. I guess my prayers were heard, for Dr. Speck arrived by horse and cutter and confirmed my suspicions. He brought the necessary equipment, and about daybreak was successful in delivering a live baby to a very weak but lucky mother. If she had stayed at home and just called in a neighbour as before, no doubt both would have died.

The other patient I mentioned was planning on being confined at home. She had seen her doctor several times and he assured her that all was well. One day I was making a routine pre-natal visit and found her in bed and hemorrhaging quite profusely. Her husband had been trying several times to reach her doctor but had not succeeded. I decided that the only logical thing to do would be to take her to Lindsay, to Ross Memorial Hospital, where a Caesarean operation could be performed if necessary. Once I explained the situation to her husband, he went back to the station and telephoned the hospital, making arrangements for a doctor to be on hand when she arrived. In the meantime, a neighbour and I made a comfortable bed for her in a large borrowed car. The doctor met us on arrival as promised and, before long, the patient was in the operating room where a Caesarean section was preformed. After the surgery the doctor told me that if she had waited much longer it would have been too late to save either her or the child. But they were both alive and well.

For some time I had been giving pre-natal advice to a woman who lived on a farm several miles away, in a very out-of-the-way place that sometimes could only be reached by team and sleigh. At first she absolutely refused to consider going to a hospital or even having a doctor. It was her first baby and she was in her late 30s, and for some reason I was worried. Finally, she consented to come to the Outpost, so late one February night her husband brought her. She was in labour, but I had a feeling it would take a long time. When morning came and nothing had happened, I was successful in convincing her that she should have a doctor. Consequently, her husband went to the store and was able to reach Dr. Lumb at Bancroft by phone in time for him to catch the train from there.

I was so thankful when he arrived, for she was having a hard time and I was sure I could not manage alone. However, this was the one day that I remember the train to be on time on its way back. At four o'clock it puffed into the station, but the stork was still a little way off! Dr. Lumb sent Aileen to the station to ask the conductor to hold the train until he was ready to go. It was about 5:30 when he left, satisfied that both mother and baby were safe.

The I.B.&O. sure had its good points! The kindness of the crew on this particular February day was only one of the many similar incidents I could mention. It is a sample of the spirit displayed by people of all walks of life in these isolated communities when someone is in trouble.

That particular episode was a fitting start for the deluge that would follow. By the end of February 1933, I had admitted five patients and four babies had been born, making a total of 106 days for this 28-day month. Any time I had for sleeping was spent on the cot in the living room, as my bed had to be used for patients.

I was extremely fortunate in having such a good housekeeper. I certainly never could have carried on as I did if it had not been for Aileen, even though she was so young and inexperienced when I arrived. She was willing to tackle anything and soon proved to be an invaluable assistant and companion. Often we had more than one patient at the Outpost at one time. In fact, once we had three mothers and three babies at the same time. During such times I hired extra help for her so that she could take over some of the simple nursing duties, especially when I had to go out on a case. The laundry at those times, of course, would be tremendous, especially with all the water having to be pumped. Often the old pump would yield only a small spurt at each laboured stroke. Then it had to be heated on the wood stove, even in

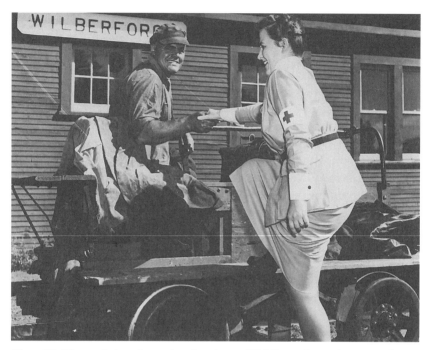

Nurse M. Chattoe being given a hand up by an I.B.&O. employee, in preparation for a ride on the rails to visit a patient circa 1950. *Courtesy Wilberforce Heritage Guild Collection.*

warm weather. But Aileen was always happy and cheerful about her work, frequently remarking that without patients to look after life would be too monotonous.

Personally, I did not find it very monotonous at any time. There was always something to be done. With all dressings having to be made and sterilized, I always tried to keep a good supply ahead, which was quite a problem at times. And there were records and reports, all of which had to be kept up-to-date. And, of course, there were clinics and school visits to plan and carry on as well as the home visiting.

Every spring a student in Public Health Nursing would be sent up from the University of Toronto for a month of fieldwork. I was supposed to see that they got as much practical experience as possible during that time. In most cases I think I succeeded. In fact, one student even had a confinement alone, without even me present. I'd had a very busy winter and spring without having a day off since Christmas, so when the student came the first of May, my supervisor suggested that I might take a weekend off, provided there were no cases expected. By the last weekend, therefore, when everything was apparently clear ahead, I left for Toronto.

Of course, that had to be the night that the old stork was flying around, so Miss Walker admitted a patient and delivered her and got along fine. But, after all, how was I to know that she would be having a baby at that particular time? Both Miss Walker and I had attended her wedding dance only three weeks before! Things do certainly happen fast in this country!

I was very thankful to have the students during the month of May, for they were able to help with the schoolwork, and so much more could be accomplished. Not only did I get the regular Public Health Nursing students, but often International Students were sent up for a few days to see the practical side of Public Health Nursing in a rural section of Canada. I had four such students at various times of the year and found them to be most interesting guests. The first, Miss Luoma, from Finland, would teach Public Health Nursing upon returning to her own country. She was finding our language quite difficult to master. Once she learned that I had kept all the notes taken during the course, she was delighted when I let her compare them with hers.

Miss Luoma had a special interest in rural homes so I took her visiting, of course not choosing the worst. I had a certain place in mind one day when we started out. To reach it we had to drive over some of the rockiest, most desolate roads in the district, as well as some of the most beautiful country. I'd had this woman as a patient at the Outpost and both she and her husband had been very friendly and cooperative. They were quite poor but very thrifty and clean. The father had made a bassinet for the new baby, which I was anxious to have my guest see. Made of thin smooth lumber, it rested on a frame of four legs on casters, with a shelf about half way down. The top was about three feet high. There was a lid to fit on the top that could be used as a table for bathing or changing the baby, but this was put aside when the bed was in use. It was all enamelled white and nicely padded inside. It pleased the mother to have us visit her and, when I explained my guest's interest in Canadian homes, she invited her to see through her whole house.

The nurse from Yugoslavia, who visited us in February, was thrilled with the snow. She had heard about snowshoes, she said, but had never seen a pair. We made sure she had a chance to try them out while she was with us. Del brought some extra ones over and we all went on a little trip, of course he didn't lead us along the smoothest trails. I can almost hear our guest now, laughing as she tried climbing the hills! I am sure she will always remember her visit to this part of Canada.

The Czechoslovakian nurse accompanied me and assisted at a home confinement without a doctor. The nurse from Romania arrived shortly after I had discharged my second pair of twins and their mother, so I took her to see them, as well as many other places which I thought would be an interest to her. We always enjoyed having the International Students,[3] and learned as much from them, I'm sure, as they did from us.

13

Midwives, Modern Methods and Home Remedies

Loving this country as I did, especially during the summer months, made me decide to ask for my three weeks vacation during the winter one year so I could spend Christmas at home with my family. Quite early on the morning of December 6th, I loaded up my coupe, taking with me as passengers a neighbour and her little girl planning to visit friends in Lindsay, a cat for my kid sister and, on top of the car, two Christmas trees. There was very little snow, but the road was a bit slippery in places, as one might expect at this time of year. But I was brave and sure that conditions would improve as we drove south-ward. We were unable to make Hadley's Hill near Gooderham with-out the help of a horse to tow us, but otherwise got along fine.

My city friends never seemed to tire of hearing about my "experi-ences away up in the wilds," and were constantly asking questions about this and that. "What did they use for medicine or in case of acci-dents when there was no doctor or nurse available, and what about childbirth, and weren't you frightened to have to attend a confinement alone?" Well to that question, "No." I was never afraid, for after all, I had received some training. And, if I were not on hand, they would have to depend on someone with no training at all. By all means, I would get a doctor if possible, but I considered that my best efforts were considerably better than the neighbour's, and the longer I was there the more I realized how much better…I also believed that it was God's will that I was there in the first place and therefore He would never forsake me as long as I kept my faith and did my best.

Seeing so many of the methods that were being used for the treatment of various illnesses, I became so used to them that nothing really surprised me, but rather made me more anxious than ever to make people aware of the services of the Red Cross. Some women, particularly those who considered themselves qualified "midwives," were a real menace to the health of the people in the community in which they lived. To call in a neighbour in case of an emergency was one thing, but to rely on these women with their cure-all remedies, not only at the same time of childbirth, but to treat other illnesses when a doctor or nurse was available, was something that many had to be taught was wrong. Some had been "practising" for a long time and were very jealous of a mere young girl taking away their glory (and fee). But as the saying goes, "Ignorance is bliss," and some took a long time to learn.

Quite often I would be called only when none of their "local" cures were successful. Sometimes the women would tell me what they had tried and, believe me, I learned a lot! For instance, boiling fresh pig lard and fresh horse manure together made a very valuable salve.[1] It was then strained into small jars and when cooled, it solidified and was used for almost everything that called for a healing salve. It was considered especially good for frostbite. Fresh cow manure alone was considered a perfect poultice for drawing out pus, slivers and other foreign bodies.

One man at camp had a very painful boil on his arm. A friend had heard that boils could be drawn out by applying hot water bottles, so undertook to fix up his chum's arm. They rinsed a bottle with very hot water and immediately placed the neck over the boil. It drew all right, but unfortunately the boil was not ready to be drawn and the misery the poor fellow went through was pitiful, until someone suggested breaking the bottle.

Poultices made of swallows' nests were supposed to cure quinsy,[2] but I've heard of a few failures. Chewing the blisters of resin from balsam trees, for some was a way to cure colds.[3] For others the soiled-sock treatment for sore throats was a common remedy.[4] Bear grease was a great cure-all, especially for chest colds and also for hair oil. One man, so the story goes, made a great mistake in using it for that purpose. He did not know that to grow hair, the oil had to be from a bear

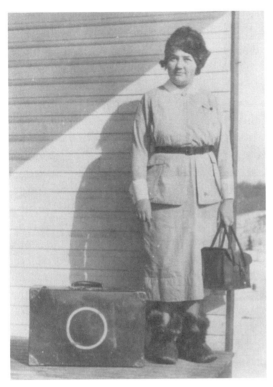

Gertrude LeRoy is on the side porch, dressed in her nurse's uniform, with the maternity kit and nurse's bag all ready to head out on a call. Galoshes were in style, but, more importantly, they kept the feet warm. *Courtesy Wilberforce Heritage Guild Collection, donated by Aileen Ames Walker.*

that was killed in the fall. This fellow's bear, unfortunately, had been killed in the spring when it was losing its hair. When he rubbed the oil into his head he had brown curly hair, but before long that hair fell out and a new crop of hair grew in, black and straight! Even I had a direct experience; I was nursing a pneumonia patient for whom Dr. Lumb prescribed bear oil instead of the usual camphorated oil to follow applications of mustard plasters.

I found, however, that the most favoured treatment for chest colds and pneumonia was onion poultices to both chest and feet. So many of the families were using this treatment that I asked one of the doctors if he thought there was any real value in it. "There certainly is," he said. "Haven't you noticed how smelly it makes the house?" He was right there!

One cold Sunday evening in January, Aileen and I were ready to leave for church when Mr. Agnew arrived with a message from Mr. S. of Harcourt. Their little girl was very ill and would I please come as soon as possible? "Yes," I said, "Tell him I'll go as soon as I can find someone to take me."

So, while I prepared myself for a seven-mile ride in an open sleigh, Aileen went across to see if Mr. White would take me. In no time she was back and said that he would pick me up in about fifteen minutes with his team and sleigh. Our destination was a nice home in the village of Harcourt. If I had gone by train it would have been about four miles, however, the road was so crooked both vertically and horizontally that it crossed the railroad tracks three times in the final two miles.

Just as we stopped at the house, we heard the put-put of a gas handcar coming from the opposite direction, then it stopped at the nearby crossing. I hurried to the house and was met at the door by the father of the sick child, whom I could hear screaming at the top of her lungs. Mr. S. ushered me into the kitchen where a roaring fire was burning in the range. The grandmother was walking the floor, trying to hold the bundled up three-year-old who was struggling and screaming. She kept talking to the child, "Now, now, my darling, here's the nurse. She will make you all better. Don't cry." The grandfather was walking up and down the room, following his wife, and also trying to console the child. The poor mother, almost beside herself, was just standing beside a carriage in which her small baby was sleeping.

Mr. S. took my wraps and I was warming my hands before going near the patient, when someone shouted, "Here's the doctor." I almost shouted for joy myself, not having known that someone had been sent to get him. Now a load rolled off my shoulders. All I would have to do now was follow orders!

Dr. Lumb, having come nearly 25 miles on the gas handcar from Bancroft, was very cold too. But soon he was warm enough to examine the child, who had not ceased her screaming. In the meantime, she had been passed from Grandma to Grandpa, then back again to Grandma. I suggested that they lay her on the table so the doctor could examine her, and I proceeded to unwrap her. Goodness, she had enough blankets around her to make a good soft bed. Finally, when I opened up the last one I found that she not only had a thick onion poultice on her chest, but her feet were tied in a bag of cooked onions as well! Poor child! No wonder she was screaming! They were sure that she had pneumonia, and Grandma said that no better cure could be found than onions, but so far they hadn't worked.

After examining the child, Dr. Lumb told the family that more than anything else, she needed to be kept quiet. He asked me if I could possibly stay for the night, or longer if necessary, in order to get her settled into a regular routine. It was not my policy to stay on cases, but

I thought that under the circumstances I might make an exception. I could easily be reached if needed elsewhere, so I sent the message back to Aileen with Mr. White.

The first thing I did for Cathy was to get her into her own bed in her own room. Dr. Lumb and I decided that it would be best that she should see no one but me. I gave her a warm sponge bath, put a mustard plaster on her chest, gave her the medicine the doctor had left. Before long she was off to dreamland, without any fuss whatever. Her parents were very co-operative from the very first, but her grandparents weren't a bit pleased about not being able to stay with her. However, when they saw how quiet she was with me, and how much better she seemed in the morning, they finally gave in and departed for their own home not far away. I stayed there for three days, at the end of which time Cathy was greatly improved and strongly objected to me leaving.

RECIPE FOR MUSTARD PLASTERS
for bronchial & chest congestion

(described by Nadeen Sanderson & Hilda Clark)

Mix 1 Tbs. dry mustard with 3 Tbs. of flour or soda.*
Add enough cold water to make a smooth paste.
Spread paste on a piece of cloth size of chest. Fold cloth over like an envelope. Place on chest for up to 15 minutes. Watch that it doesn't burn, i.e. skin turning red. Remove and cover chest with some warm material such as flannel. Repeat later if necessary.

*Soda helps prevent burning.

One winter, road work was being done at a rock cut quite near the home of one of my "rivals" in the Maternity Department. Naturally she was making what money she could by boarding several of the workmen. One evening I received a message that a man had been injured very seriously. That was all the information I had. The only possible way I could go was by gas car, which would take me about 1½ miles from the home where I would find the patient. The section man took me and it wasn't very long until we were at the station. Not seeing anyone there, I went up to the store from where the message had been sent, sure that someone would be waiting with some kind of conveyance, but no such luck. I learned from the storekeeper that a man had come in and called Dr. Frain. The doctor was not sure he could make the trip because of snowdrifts, so had advised him to send for me, just in case he couldn't get through. He would have to come by horse and cutter and change horses half way. Immediately after making the calls, the man had left, leaving no message for me.

The only thing left for me to do was to pick up my bag and walk. I knew it was well over a mile and I wasn't looking forward to trudging through the snow up and down the hills that lay ahead. My bag got heavier and heavier as I pushed on through the drifts. Fortunately, there was a little moonlight, since my flashlight wasn't of much use. I didn't mind the cold as I was getting enough exercise to keep warm.

According to the information given by the storekeeper, the victim had been struck in the back by a rock when they were blasting. He understood that the man was quite badly injured.

Finally, I saw the light at the farmhouse and my bag seemed to get a little lighter and my heart started beating a little faster. I was not looking forward to an encounter with this woman in her own home. Goodness only knew what treatment or remedy she'd have used by this time. No doubt she would resent my having been called, and she did!

I knocked on the door and the lady herself opened it. "Well!" she said, "It took you long enough to get here."

"Yes," I said. "It's quite a walk from the station. How is the patient?"

"He's just as good as can be expected," she said, emphasizing every word. She made no move to take my coat, but her husband very kindly suggested that I take off my things and come over to the stove and get warm.

When I asked to see the patient, she said, "Well, I think he's asleep but I'll take you in. I gave him a good dose of coal oil (kerosene). There's nothing like coal oil when it comes to a sore back. He didn't like the idea of taking it but I finally got it down him and I'm sure he's the better for it. The men insisted on sending for the doctor but I didn't see any sense in it. I don't think there is anything you can do."

All this talk and we hadn't yet reached the patient's room. Perhaps he wasn't as severely injured as I had been led to believe. Just as we reached the bedroom door, her husband called from the kitchen, "Min, here's the doctor!"

What wonderful words! He had really come! Thank goodness! I

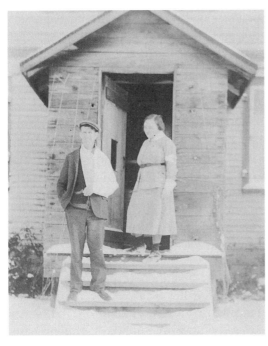

Gertrude LeRoy discharging a patient from the Outpost. *Courtesy Wilberforce Heritage Guild Collection, donated by the Schofield family.*

helped as he examined the patient, who complained of a considerable amount of pain. The doctor could detect no broken bones and decided quiet rest in bed was the best treatment. He certainly was not very pleased about the coal oil treatment, but said he didn't think it had done him any harm. He had me give the patient a shot of morphine to ease the pain and left me some tablets with written instructions, to be given later. After the doctor and I had done all we could for the patient, the hostess actually made us a cup of tea! No doubt she realized that we had no intention of stealing her patient, so she might as well be friendly.

One very cold December day I received a message that there was a very sick patient in Kennaway. Would I please come at once. Although it was mid-winter, there was very little snow in spite of the cold and I was still driving my car, so I wasted no time. My destination, about a mile from Kennaway School where Hazel [Miller] was teaching, was set on the shore of a fair-sized lake. I found the patient upstairs in bed, writhing in pain. A neighbour, Mrs. C. was there doing what she thought was best to ease her pain, applying heat by means of a hot iron wrapped in towels. I suspected appendicitis and immediately changed the treatment, and told the patient that a doctor must be sent for at once. She said she couldn't possibly do that. Her husband was out on his trapline, she said, and she would not send for a doctor unless he said to do so. I dispatched the eldest boy to find his father and tell him to come home at once. It seemed hours to me and no doubt much longer to the patient, before her husband arrived, out of breath. Once I explained the seriousness of the situation to him, he immediately sent his son to Harcourt on horseback to telephone for a doctor.

I felt absolutely useless in the meantime, as there was so little I could do, but finally Dr. Frain arrived. After examining the patient, he asked me, "What do you think is wrong?"

"You know that nurses do not diagnose," I replied.

"Forget you're a nurse," he said, "Tell me what you think."

"It looks like appendicitis to me," I said.

"I'm sure that's what it is, but I can't very well operate here. Anyway, I'm afraid she is going to die. If I operate here and she should die, people would no doubt blame me for her death. And I'm afraid she couldn't stand the trip to Lindsay, or even to Haliburton. No matter where she is, if she lives, she is going to require a lot of good care. Something must be done at once, so what do you think of moving her to the Outpost? We'll see how well she stands it that far, and perhaps I'll operate there."

I assured him that I would certainly agree with anything he should decide to do. So he went downstairs and talked to the family. He told them of his fears and asked the husband what his wishes were. He said by all means take her to the Outpost if she would have a better chance of recovery.

In the meantime Hazel arrived from her boarding place and offered her help. As this was Friday, she could go back to Wilberforce with me. As quickly as we could we made the back of the doctor's car into a bed, using a large feather tick, pillows and quilts. He had me give the patient a fairly large dose of morphine and, when she was settled as comfortable as possible in that car, Hazel and I struck out in mine. Her husband accompanied the doctor and patient. I paid little attention to the hard frozen ruts and bumps in the road, my object being to get to the Outpost as soon as possible to prepare for an operation, which was something very unusual.

With Aileen's help, much was accomplished by the time the doctor arrived with the patient. They had had to drive much more carefully. Before attempting to move her, Dr. Frain checked the patient and found that she had stood the trip very well and was much brighter and had little pain. Perhaps she should be taken right on, at least to Haliburton, where another doctor was available. When he returned inside, he said he had decided to continue on.

Later I learned that when they arrived in Haliburton, well after midnight, the patient's condition encouraged them to take her on to Lindsay on the 4:30 a.m. train. There, in a real hospital with expert surgeons, she was successfully operated on for ruptured appendix, and in due time was back home, well and happy.

The next summer this family moved eight miles further from civilization into Bruton Township where the husband was put in charge of the fire tower. They had not been there long when I received a message, relayed from the fire tower, that one of their girls was very ill. They were bringing her by boat, as far as their old home in Kennaway, and asked to have me meet them there and bring her back to the Outpost.

I set out immediately. When I arrived at the lakeshore I could see a canoe coming down the lake with, what I thought, were two passengers in it. However, as it drew near I could see a third person lying on the bottom. Myrtle was dreadfully swollen and I could tell she had a high temperature. Her mother and uncle were with her and they told me they'd had to walk four miles, then come four miles by canoe. The mother said she was putting Myrtle completely in my care, and wished me to do whatever I thought best. Send for the doctor if I thought it was necessary.

Poor Myrtle was pretty well exhausted by the time we reached the Outpost. I put her to bed and began irrigating her throat with a salt and soda solution as warm as she could stand it. I was sure it was a case of quinsy (abscessed tonsils), so I repeated these irrigations regularly throughout the night. Quite early the next morning the abscess broke, her temperature went down and she began to feel much better.

While she was with us, the annual Red Cross Picnic was held and we took her to see the sights. Myrtle was 14 years old and had never seen many people, and certainly never attended such a large picnic. Well, she would have plenty to tell her folks when she went home! How we did enjoy seeing her eat ice cream! Evidently it was the first time she had tasted it. She was wishing she could take some home for her sister.

One afternoon I took her over to Haliburton. I wanted Dr. Frain to check her over before she had to go on the four-mile hike home. That was another outing she enjoyed. I had Mr. Agnew send a message through to the tower and we reversed the procedure of the previous week, a trip which I'm sure she found more pleasant.

One evening an eight month-old child was brought to the Outpost by his parents who lived on a farm several miles away. One look at him told me that he was a very sick child. He was so emaciated and weak that he could not hold his head up. They told me that he had been very cross for weeks, and would sleep only when they walked the floor with him. They had taken him to Dr. Frain a few days ago and he had explained that the baby needed a change of food. He had given them some sour tasting stuff which was "not fit for a pig," so the mother had thrown it out. Now the parents had come to see what I could suggest.

I realized that no matter what I suggested, she would perhaps do the same. After thinking the matter over carefully, I suggested that they leave the baby with me for a while. I said it would give me a chance to get him started on a formula that would agree with him. It took a lot of persuasion, but finally they consented and left without him.

I'd had great success with a butter soup formula, which I had seen used for undernourished infants at the Hospital for Sick Children, so I made up some for Johnny. Made of flour, butter, sugar, water and milk, the mixture had many more calories per ounce than regular milk feedings. The poor child was starving and took it without any coaxing.

We put the crib in my room so I could look after him during the night. I then bathed him and put him to bed. That was when the fun started! He began to cry, and I remembered what the parents had told me about taking turns walking the floor with him every night, so I picked him up and started to walk. Sure enough, he stopped crying and closed his eyes. I put him back into the bed and he really did yell at the top of his lungs. I picked him up again and walked back and forth across the room a couple of times and he was off to dreamland again. So down he went once more, this time to stay in spite of his screams! Cruel woman! I was glad his parents couldn't hear him, but I realized the sooner the matter was settled the better for both of us. He cried for quite a while, then settled down to sleep, until 6 a.m.

The next day I was able to get in touch with Dr. Frain and explained about the feedings. He laughed when I told him what had become of his formula. He advised me to carry on as I was doing and to let him know he said, should some help be needed. I had done the wise thing in keeping the baby there, and suggested that I add vegetables to his diet.

Well, that night we went through the same performance and, as soon as I was sure that he was comfortable, I just let him cry. This time it was not quite so long until he fell asleep. The third night the crying time was shortened considerably, and from then on he just went to sleep as soon as he was tucked in.

Johnny began to pick up and was soon strong enough to sit up alone. At the end of two weeks, when his parents came for him, he was creeping, had gained two pounds and had cut two teeth! Needless to say, the parents were delighted. Of course, I had kept them informed of his progress.

Mrs. X, who called herself a midwife and attended most of the women in her neighbourhood when they had their babies, had some very queer ideas about caring for the babies as well as the mothers. One time, when her system failed, I was called to a home about eight miles away. When I arrived, Mrs. X was there with the mother and both were very upset about the condition of her three-week-old baby. As soon as I saw it I was sure it was dying. In spite of all my efforts, he could not be revived.

Mrs. X told me that she had delivered Mrs. S. three weeks before and noticed that the baby was very delicate. She was sure the mother's milk was not strong enough, so had advised her not to nurse the baby but feed him a mixture of cream and water. He did not start to gain so she had given him a few doses of soot (from the stovepipe)! The poor baby died.

Another woman ordered supplementary feedings of fresh cow's milk for a new baby. Every time the baby was to be fed, someone had to go to the stable and get a few ounces of milk from the cow and, without diluting it, give it to the baby while it was warm.

I found that some woman relied on untrained midwives for the simple reason that their mothers and grandmothers had done it and so, why should they need better now? And there was another reason that shocked me more. A woman who was expecting her 15th baby was advised to have the nurse or doctor rather than the usual neighbour. She said she'd had neither doctor or nurse when she had the other 14 and, if she were to have one this time, it wouldn't be fair to the others.

What shocked me most of all, however, was to learn that some women didn't even have the assistance of a neighbour, the husband being the only attendant. I guess those husbands thought that since they were capable of attending the cows and sheep when they had their young, they were just as capable of attending their wives at such times, for, after all, wasn't it just a natural process? And why should he give $5 to a nurse or $25 to a doctor when he could manage everything himself?

One woman whom I was attending told me how lucky she felt to have a nurse when she was having her baby. She said her mother, who lived in another part of the county, had given birth to ten children. Always when her time came, she would send one of the children to the field for her husband. He would come in, attend to her and, when everything was over, he would go back to his work in the field. (No doubt he didn't even wash his hands in the process). Well, perhaps that system worked out all right ten times, but not long after that I heard that the mother died when giving birth to her eleventh child.

Considering the number of obstetrical cases I had attended since my arrival in Wilberforce, it looked as if the Red Cross was winning over the local "midwives". It so happened, too, that two of the so-called "midwives" had to call on the Red Cross Nurse to save their own lives.

The first incident happened in the winter when, in answer to a telephone message, Sid White's team had to fight deep snowbanks to get me there. In the process the cutter upset. When we finally arrived, a neighbour of the patient met me at the door and very excitedly urged me to hurry, as something was wrong. One glance was all I needed to tell me what the trouble was, for the baby's head was exposed and was almost black. The umbilical cord was looped around the infant's neck, choking it and preventing it from being born. Fortunately, I was able to loosen the cord and slip it over the head without cutting it. Once the head was freed, the child was born without any more difficulty. After working over it for a few minutes, the baby finally gave a good healthy cry. I was quite sure it would be all right. This was the first time I had been confronted with such a situation, but I had learned about such cases during training.

The other case was during a more pleasant time of year, but it meant a very fast eighteen-mile drive late at night. When I arrived, the baby had been born and apparently well looked after, but the mother was in an almost hysterical state and bleeding profusely. Only her husband was present. He said he had been managing very well under his wife's directions, but the afterbirth wouldn't come away and his wife couldn't tell him what to do. Practically everything around was saturated with blood.

I immediately made an attempt to massage her abdomen, but she protested and forbade me to touch her. When she persisted, I pretended I was about to leave. "Well," I said, "Since you know more about this sort of thing than I do, I might as well go home. Too bad your husband bothered to send for me. At the rate you are hemorrhaging, you haven't much longer to live, if that's what you want." I knew I had to say something that would bring her to her senses, as I didn't want to have to use force.

It did have the desired effect. "Please, Nurse, don't leave me," she begged. "Do what you have to do." I went right to work and in a very short time the placenta was expelled and uterus contracted and bleeding eased off. I stayed with her until I was sure her condition was satisfactory. When I left, her attitude toward me had changed considerably and we became good friends. She decided that her "midwife" days were over.

14

The Cottage and a Tale of Scouts

Needless to say, I was certainly falling in love with these "Haliburton Highlands," and so was every member of my family. Mother visited me during the winter and liked it even then. I began thinking how nice it would be if I owned a cottage where they could come whenever they wished. The more I thought of it the better I liked the idea. Early in the spring of 1933, after I had finished paying for my car, I began looking around for a suitable site to have one built. I was talking the matter over with Del one Sunday afternoon and he said, "Why not look at my grandfather's[1] old place at South Wilberforce?"

"Where is it?" I asked.

"About 4½ miles down the road toward Tory Hill, on the right just as you cross the second bridge."

I had travelled that way often, but the road was so crooked in that area that I was watching the road rather than scenery. Consequently, I hadn't paid much attention to the house, except to know it was empty. I did recall having noticed an old picket fence bordering the road.

"That was it," he said, "And now it belongs to my Uncle Joe[2] who lives on the next farm." He was quite sure his uncle would sell it. The house hadn't been occupied for some time and would no doubt need

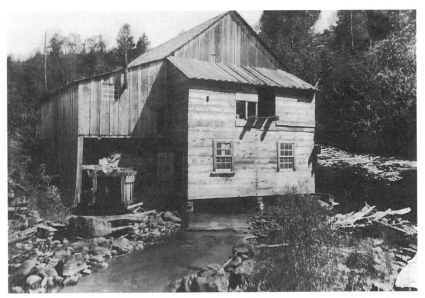

This sawmill, built and operated by Richard Dunford, maternal grandfather of A'Delbert Miller, sat beside the river near the "Cottage" that Gertrude LeRoy purchased in 1933. *Courtesy Wilberforce Heritage Guild Collection, donated by Jim Deterling.*

some repairs, but it was a very well-built house. He suggested that we go and look at it anyways, so off we went.

On the way he told me about his grandfather having a sawmill [3] at the falls just below the house, and that he had built the house in the early 1890s. Around that area had been the original settlement of Wilberforce, before the railroad went through to the north.

An earlier chapter Isabel Shay told a bit about the original settlement, and even about the house.[4] Now, as we approached it, the house seemed to be in a rather delapidated condition, especially the floor of the porch, which extended across the front and south side. Of course we couldn't see too much through the windows, but it surely could be fixed up, at least good enough for a summer place.

As we turned to leave, I looked around at the scenery and gasped! It was beautiful in every direction: the lake, the river, the hills, the rocks and the trees! I decided right then and there that if the place were for sale and at a price within my means, I would certainly buy it.

Before going over to his uncle's for the key, Del suggested that we walk down along the river so he could show me where his grandfather had his mill. As we picked our way through the brush we could hear the exciting musical sound of a waterfall. Finally we came out to the edge of the gorge, a high wall of rocks on the far side. Several feet below a shallow stream rushed past, through piles of driftwood and sunken logs. Farther on we came to the old dam which had been partially washed out, and down below was the old mill pond, with the forsaken water wheel lying on the bottom among the pieces of driftwood. On the shore were a couple of rotted-down piles of slabs. Climbing the hill, we followed the river as it meandered along, dividing here and there to form small islands, some growing beautiful cedars. In fact, these cone-shaped trees were everywhere, as well as pines, balsams, spruce and the beautiful white birch.

So we went over to see Uncle Joe. Yes, he would sell the place. Besides the house, there were sixteen acres of land! About three acres around the house were cleared. The rest formed a strip along the river. It included some swampland containing softwood and also a small sugar bush. I figured that the price he asked was very reasonable compared to what I would have to pay for a lot and have a cottage built. And the scenery here couldn't possibly be matched! I didn't hesitate to close the deal.[5]

Although it was a two-story building, wc always rcfcrrcd to it as thc "Cottage." Since I was too busy at the Outpost to have much time to spend fixing up the place, I just let my family carry on. They really got back to nature during the summers. After bringing up odds and ends of furniture and lots of friends, they really enjoyed themselves. I was delighted to have them so nearby. We helped them plant a garden, which provided them with lots of fresh vegetables. The lake produced all the fish they could eat.

That year the Red Cross Picnic was held in August. My brother-in-law[6] brought his Boy Scout Troop which put on a Minstrel Show to help raise funds for the Red Cross. That was really something, as I'm sure none of the locals had ever seen anything like it. It was just as exciting for the Scouts, since the majority of them had never been so far from the city, and certainly never in such surroundings as those in which they pitched their tents. The spot they chose was right beside the falls on the old millstream on my land.

When they returned home, a report of their adventures was written for their bulletin by Pete Saunders, one of the troop. Only quotations from it can give a fair account of their reactions:

"Away back in the winter the rumor started to get around. The Minstrel Show is going to Wilberforce. Immediately the question arose, "Who, what, when, and where is Wilberforce?" When, with the help of maps and geographies, we finally found out that it was a

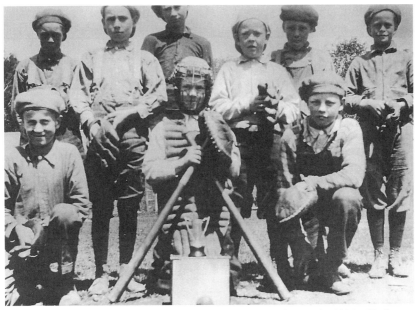

Likely this hardball team played at a Red Cross Picnic, circa early 1930s. Back row (l to r): Art Fleming, Elgin Bowen, Herbert Barker, Gerald Rose, Bill Clark, Frank Minns. Front row: Ken White, Duard Rose, Vince Godfrey. *Courtesy Hilda Clark Collection.*

little village in the back woods about one hundred and sixty miles northeast of Toronto, it seemed beyond possibility that we city slickers should ever get there.

"However, a certain fortunate five of us were one day asked rather tentatively what we thought of the idea. The answer was so enthusiastic that 'Cap' had to caution us to keep it under cover and not to anticipate too much.

"Well, when things were finally settled, it appeared that the Thirtieth Toronto Troop Minstrel Show (the immortal MacNamara Special) was going to be produced on the evening of the Wilberforce Red Cross Outpost's Field Day, August 5th, 1933. The cast (the gang) was to come up by car and what have you, on the Field Day. It seems that the aforementioned fortunate five were to go up with Don LeRoy on July 29th and camp for the week preceeding the show. The five were George Robinson, Jim McLeod, Fred Clark, Star Stamp, and Pete Saunders. Were we feeling our oats? Not half! Just imagine going camping in the great north country! Not really as far as Kirkland Lake, but at least almost as far as Algonquin Park!

"The big day finally arrived and after hastily gathering up the last minute things, the chariot set sail and pulled out from Stamp's at half past twelve. Most of our equipment, tents and grub had gone ahead on the train, we hoped. After later having a look at the train, we certainly considered ourselves lucky that it got there.

"Don appeared rather quiet at first, but we soon broke down his reserve. If five scouts out for a holiday can't get under a fellow's skin, then he is certainly a deaf mute, especially after having two flat tires.

"After leaving Fenelon Falls we struck a very dusty single track road and unfortunately were just behind a car load of women. They simply tore along at twenty miles an hour, and although women always come first, our thoughts were far from courteous. It was ninety in the shade that day, too. Until we passed them at Irondale, our idea of the country was a little hazy, but when we came out of the haze we saw that we had really reached the sticks. Most of the country was wooded and the road was just a pair of wheel tracks, often with grass growing between them. Bedrock formed the road (so called) in places, and in others it was old corduroy road covered with mud. One could easily imagine our ancestors, with all their household goods piled in an old wagon, plodding along toward greener fields.

"Just at dusk we pulled into LeRoy's 'Cottage' and were thankful for an invitation to supper. We got the tent up, and after supper prowled

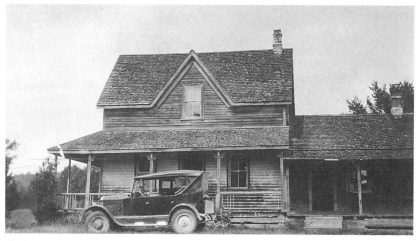

A vintage car sits in front of Gertrude's "Cottage." When she married A'Delbert Miller, it became their permanent home. *Courtesy Wilberforce Heritage Guild Collection, donated by Gerald and Bessie Shackleton, who purchased the house from Gertrude in 1974.*

around a little to get the lay of the land. We were camped near an old mill, practically demolished, on a river leading out of a lake on the other side of the road. Our tent was pitched on nice velvety grass on a slight rise. We learned that we were about four miles from Wilberforce, and it certainly looked as if we were a hundred miles from nowhere!

"We were very glad to hit the hay that night until we discovered the identity of the 'hay'. It was about one inch of turf broken at frequent intervals by sharp points of bedrock. Surprising what Wilberforce air does for you. After a week of that we looked like living corkscrews, but that just gave us a rustic appearance and we got along better with the inhabitants.

"Del Miller was our friend and guide during our stay, and he certainly proved to be a fine fellow, both as friend and guide. We spent the week preceeding the big show getting to know the country, and what a country! Imagine going fishing and really catching fish, even enough for a meal. Early in the week we made our first trip to Wilberforce proper, on our way to the crystal mine. We wore uniforms to make a good impression on the town, but after walking all day in the woods we decided that uniforms is not the thing for the bush. That day we visited Cedar Lake, the crystal mine, and a muskrat farm, as well as Mr. and Mrs. Hornet and all their friends and relatives. The average was four hornet stings each, not bad for amateurs. On that hike we were first introduced to the world renowned Trapper's Tea. Mr. Miller poured, ably assisted by Don LeRoy, beautifully gowned in a pair of "grads". Mr. Miller was using his new tea set. The glint of the tin pail in the sun was enchantingly reflected from the baked bean tin used as a cup. It was passed around from hand to hand, thus reviving the old English custom of the Wassail bowl. A new recipe was used to make the tea, and we thought that you might like to use it at your next social event. To one tin pail of lake water add one pound of tea, any brand, let boil over a smokey hot fire with lots of ashes falling in the top. When a spoon will stand up in the solution unaided it is ready to serve. Serve in a bean or soup can with ragged edge. You will find that a dash of maple syrup gives it the right tang. Do not serve with cream or sugar. Your guests will drink at least two, probably three cans of this delicious beverage. (We did).

"On Saturday, August 5th, the rest of the crowd, 'Cap' and Reta,[7] Laurie and Dorothy, Len and Wink, Bert Holliday, Jimmy Pallette, Al Kidd, Lloyd Brownridge, and Bruce Henderson arrived with vulgar city customs and slick stories of how they were going to show us old woodsmen the way to fish.

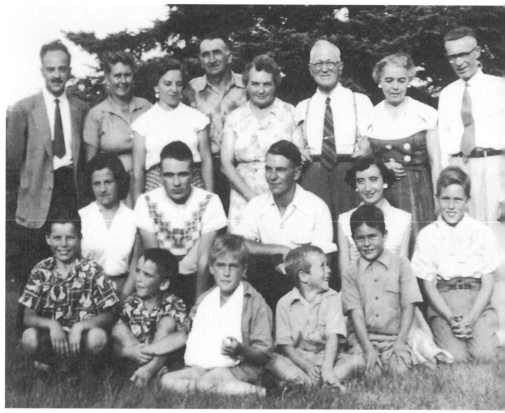

A LeRoy family gathering at Gert and Del Miller's house. Back row: (left to right) Don LeRoy and wife Lillice LeRoy; Virginia LeRoy Luckock; Del Miller; Gertrude LeRoy Miller; Charles LeRoy (Gert's father); Reta LeRoy Keay and husband Stewart "Cap" Keay. Middle row: Gloria Luckock; Gerald (Dick) Miller; Melville Miller; Lorna Keay; Rod LeRoy. Front row: Douglas Luckock; Cam Luckock; Bob LeRoy; John LeRoy and Alex LeRoy. *Courtesy Virginia LeRoy Luckock Collection*

"That night the big event of the year finally hit town in the one and only public hall.[8] What suspense before the curtain was pulled to show those dusky faces straight from Alabam'! How they shone in the light of the Coleman lamps (advt.), how those sweet voices rang out over the dense throng of excited folks in their Sunday best! The gang put on a real show, and according to comments afterwards, everyone enjoyed it to the utmost.

"The next morning (Sunday), Del arrived bright and early (too early for most of them thar city slickers) and took us up to Grace Lake. It was a beautiful place, set down in the hills like an amethyst on green

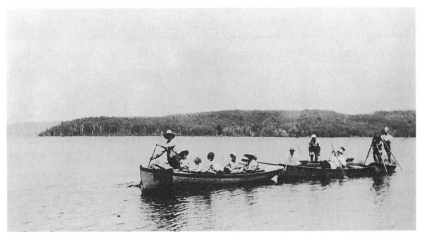

Boating on Grace Lake circa early 1930s. *Courtesy Wilberforce Heritage Guild Collection*

velvet. However, the swimming was more important than the scenery and we took advantage of it. On the way back Del decided to show us some bush, so we plunged right in and fought our way through bush and brambles for a couple of hours. In the end we found out that we were about twenty feet from a well-beaten trail all the time!

"That afternoon we all donned our uniforms and attended church in a body. The minister was so pleased, he changed his sermon to suit the occasion. On returning, a few of the fortunate five went out and caught all the fish that were needed for supper. Isaac Walton Muir, who had fished all morning and managed to catch one bass, will never get over it. He still thinks we bought them.

"Monday morning we went to visit the mink ranch (which gave the girls expensive ideas) and also visited the balancing rock. This is a huge rock standing on the edge of a cliff and balancing on a small point. About eleven of us stood on it at once.

"At noon the gang pulled out, leaving Fred Clark, Al Kidd, and Pete Saunders to hold the fort. The idea being that there wasn't enough car space to take everybody and we were unlucky enough to be left behind (oh yeah). We were supposed to be taken home at the end of the week, but actually it was another week after that before we weighed anchor. Were we sorry? Not much!

"We really pioneered during that week and a half. For days we didn't go to town or see anybody. One-day Del's brother, Geordie, took us on a promised trip to Yangton Lake. Del had been telling us about it ever since we had come to Wilberforce. It was really worth telling about. Del had a hunting shack there and several boats. He also had a birch bark canoe which Fred and Peter tried out. Fred has now decided that, to get into a canoe, you do not reach across and grasp the opposite gunwale. His lovely plus fours were slightly dampened much to his disgust. To those who haven't tried it, let me say that a birch bark canoe with one person in it in a brisk breeze is second cousin to a merry go around.

"Fred, Al, and Pete will never die from cancer, at least they shouldn't. Geordie took us up to the radium mine one day and we each had a drink of radium water on the house. The mine wasn't working just then, so we explored it ourselves and had quite a thrilling time blundering around in the dark, trying to save our flashlights. All the ore is sent to Germany to be processed and there is very little radium in a ton of ore.

"On the last day we decided to get up early and go fishing in order to have something to take home. Just as we got nicely started there was a downpour that nearly sank the boat, and certainly made us look like fish.

"We never did know whether the LeRoys noticed their garden when they came back, but we lived for a week and a half at a dollar and a half each, so figure it out!"9

15

Putting Down Roots
While Moving On

Isabel McEwen, the new Nursing Superintendent, visited us early in
the spring of 1934 and told me some plans that were underfoot at
Headquarters. They would like me to go to Bancroft, where I would
be in charge of a much larger Outpost. I would have two nurses working under me and I was to organize a Public Health Program similar
to the one we had here.

The idea about floored me! Naturally I felt quite honored to have
them think I was capable of such an undertaking. But move away from
Wilberforce after buying the "Cottage!" Anyway, Delbert had finally
persuaded me he was the person with whom I should settle down, and
we were making plans to be married in the fall. We thought it best not
to tell anyone for the time being. However, there were many factors to
consider and many other reasons I could think of for refusing. The one
I finally gave Miss McEwen, however, and meant it very sincerely, was
that, in my opinion, a Public Health Program in an area such as Bancroft would require a full-time Public Health Nurse. Knowing how busy
they were kept with their three nurses now, the charge nurse would certainly have little time for outside duties. Also, I was not interested in
doing straight hospital duty. She was quite understanding and said that
at the present time the Red Cross could not afford to hire an extra nurse.

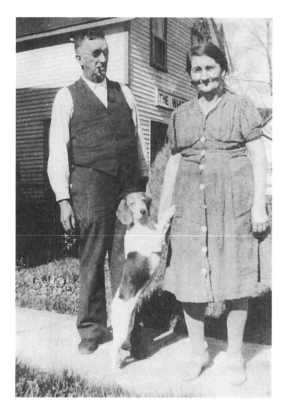

George and Melissa (Dunford) Miller, A'Delbert's parents. Mrs. Miller often looked after Gertrude and Delbert's sons when Gertrude would be called back in to serve at the Outpost Hospital.

So that was settled and, incidently, Bancroft did not get a Public Health Nurse until 1967.

In spite of the Depression, we decided to get married early in September and set about making plans for the future. Of course I would have to give up my job. There was no place in the nursing profession for married women in those days, as there was a great surplus of unmarried nurses. And where would we live? There was one small three-room cottage in town available to rent or buy but neither of us liked it. But what about the "Cottage?" It was four miles from town, but we had the car so Del could drive to work. Instead of paying rent we would fix it up. There were neighbours fairly close by, so I shouldn't be lonely. We could grow our own vegetables and possibly raise a pig or two to provide pork. And, naturally, everybody kept a cow to provide milk, cream and butter, so we would be no different.

But now it was spring with all its usual spring activities, visits to the schools and other duties as soon as the roads dried up a bit. But it was usually about April before one could be sure of not getting stuck in the mud. There were two home confinements in April, one being a very difficult one in Cheddar. Fortunately, we were able to get Dr. Lumb to come from Bancroft, and both mother and baby came through the ordeal, safe and sound.

There were only two confinements during May and June. It seemed that the old stork was taking a rest or had moved to parts unknown. I soon found out, however, that it had just been resting up in order to make its final thrust at me! On July 14th I began wearing my solitaire,[1] and announced that I would be leaving the Outpost in the fall. BANG! That did it! Starting July 15th and during the next four weeks, eight babies were born, including one pair of twins! And I had all the cases alone except two, when a doctor officiated. And only one confinement took place at the Outpost, which meant that I had to travel many miles every day to give bedside care.

The case I attended at the Outpost involved a very exciting race with the stork. After receiving a message to go to Hadlington, an old ghost settlement in the southernmost part of the county, I struck out as fast as I could on the very crooked 15 mile drive. I had been with this patient three years before when she had her first baby, so realized her second one would undoubtedly come much faster. I arrived to find the patient fully dressed and walking the floor. Her pains were coming quite fast, she said, so I began to unpack my equipment.

"Oh, no!" she shouted, "I'm not staying here! I want you to take me to the Outpost!"

"We may not have time to get there," I said. "This baby will not take as long as your first one did and it's a long drive."

"I don't care," she said. "I would rather have it on the road than stay back here! I just have to go!"

So, with her sister's help, we finally got her and all the luggage into the car and away we went! But what would I be able to do in a little Ford Coupe if the stork should overtake us? Fifteen miles to go, over rough roads! Should I go slowly and easily over the bumps, or go fast and hope for the best? I chose the latter.

As I have already mentioned, the road for the first eight miles from Hadlington was very narrow and very, very crooked. But worst of all, there was not one house along the way. After that, the main road was not quite so crooked but rougher with more hills. However, here and there all the rest of the way were houses where we could seek help if necessary. The patient kept urging me to hurry, so I did! I saw some men working on a section of the road some distance ahead, so I just pressed on the horn to warn them to get out of the way, as well as pressing on the accelerator. The men stood on the side of the road and stared at us as we passed, wondering, I suppose, where the fire was! I am sure none of them had ever seen or heard an ambulance, but they were seeing one then!

When we stopped at the Outpost we were still ahead of the stork. Aileen was at hand to help us get moved into the room and, before long, all preparations were completed. I actually had a few minutes to sit down and catch my breath. I let Aileen get the crib ready to receive the new baby, and soon a wee baby girl arrived. As soon as I was sure she was all right I wrapped her up and called Aileen to come and get her. She had just nicely tucked the baby in and returned to the kitchen, when she heard me call again. She came hurrying to the door, thinking something was wrong. But there wasn't; I just put another baby girl into her arms! Aileen was so excited she could hardly hold her! What if this had happened on the road?

As usual, there were many other duties to perform besides delivering babies that last August, but two tragic incidents marred our spirits. I was attending the babies one afternoon when word came that Dr. Frain had died! He had gone swimming with some friends at a summer resort near Haliburton and suffered a heart attack.[2] What a shock! I had lost a wonderful friend upon whom I had learned to depend so much. I was glad I would not be working at the Outpost much longer, now that he was gone. Many people would sadly miss him.

Shortly after that, tragedy also struck another home, about fifteen miles away. A little boy had picked up his father's loaded .22 rifle and accidently shot his younger sister. I was sent for immediately. A doctor, who was camping nearby, heard the accident and arrived about the same time, but she died a few minutes later.

On August 31st, I turned everything over to my successor and set out for Toronto with some of my family who had been staying at the cottage. Del and I were married the following week and after a brief honeymoon, settled down on our little "farm." I thought my nursing days were over. Actually, they were, until a week before Christmas, when the new nurse (the second one since I'd left) came down to ask me to relieve her so she could go home for the holiday. She would leave on the train Friday, the day before Christmas, so there would be nothing to do. (I had heard similar statements before so did not put much faith in that).

Of course we had made plans of our own for our first Christmas, but we realized that the nurse was lonely and a long way from home. My first Christmas at Wilberforce had been very busy and with no one to relieve me, I had not even thought of going home.

By this time we had a cow, which had to be milked every morning and night and, as Del was working every day, he would have to come home to a cold house and prepare his own meals and do the chores. Fortunately, we'd been having good weather and very little snow so far, so it was still possible to get around by car. Del said he would be able to manage for those four days. (Knowing this country and the train service and possibility of snowstorms, we secretly figured six days). So I consented to relieve her and was there when she left on the train that Friday afternoon.

Christmas turned out to be a beautiful day. As there were no patients we were able to enjoy a lovely Christmas dinner at the Millers.[3] I had

A copy of Gertrude and A'Delbert's marriage certificate indicates that they were married at St. Columba's (United) Church in Toronto on September 8, 1934. Witnesses were Gert's sister, Reta Keay and brother-in-law Stewart Keay. *With permission of Gerald R. Miller and the Miller family.*

175

no calls out and was hoping for a quiet day or two before going home, but Mr. Stork found out I was in town and on the job! Early the next morning, December 26th, a young couple drove in from out of town. I knew them well. She was expecting her first baby, though not for another month. She had been having pains all night so had called the doctor. He advised her to come to the Outpost and he would come right away.

I proceeded to prepare her for delivery and had to make it snappy, for the baby was wasting no time, and did arrive ahead of the doctor. To my horror, the moment I saw it I realized there was something wrong. During my training I had seen several cases of spina bifida and knew without a doubt that this was such a case. How I hoped it would start to breath! Should I try to make her breath? I did not have to wonder long, for she gave a good healthy cry, with no help from me! The mother was fine and, of course, having had no anaesthetic knew all that went on. I told her that her baby was a girl, and when she asked if it was all right I thought it best to tell her the truth. I told her I was afraid there was something wrong with her back, but the doctor would be here shortly and would explain after he examined her.

Well, that was December 26th, the day of the worst snowstorm of the winter. It was snowing a little when Dr. Speck arrived in his car, but was coming down much faster by the time he was ready to leave. I learned later that he had only gone about seven miles when he had to abandon his car and get a farmer to drive him the rest of the way by horse and cutter.

With all that snow, I hardly expected the nurse to return on Monday as she had promised. Well, she didn't, nor did she come Wednesday, the next train day! But a letter did arrive, saying that she had decided to stay until after New Years! She hoped I didn't mind. Well I did mind, but there was nothing I could do but stay on at the Outpost. With all the snow now, Del had to abandon the use of the car and so had a long walk to work, all the more reason I should be at home when he arrived home. However, I was finding plenty to keep me busy here. The nurse had certainly chosen a fine time to take a holiday! While she was away I not only had that one confinement at the Outpost, but two others in their homes, both without a doctor! One was a first baby and a very difficult breech delivery. Also, the supply of dressings was used up and had to be replenished.

The nurse finally returned the first train day after New Year, and indeed I was ready to leave when the train arrived. Since our next

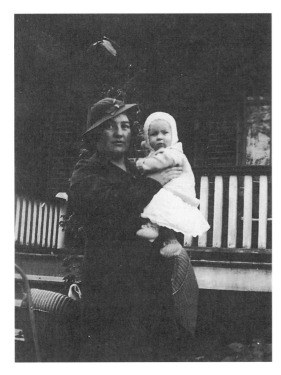

Gertrude LeRoy Miller with infant son, Melville. *Courtesy Virginia LeRoy Luckock Collection.*

door neighbour had come to town with team and sleigh to get the mail, he would take me home. In about an hour we pulled up at our front door. You can imagine my surprise to be confronted by two large signs, "WANTED—A COOK" and "NO NURSE NEED APPLY."

I relieved the nurse again a short time later, while she accompanied an accident victim to a Toronto hospital, but this time it was very peaceful and she was only gone from one train day to the next. In April she called on me to assist her at a confinement in the neighbourhood. The doctor had been called but bad roads made it impossible for him to make the trip. It was a very difficult case, however we managed very well and the mother and the baby got along all right.

Early in May I had a very thrilling experience in the form of a small parcel I received by registered mail from Government House, Toronto. Included was a letter from H.A. Bruce, Lieutenant-Governor, which said, "I have the pleasure in herewith sending you King George Fifth's Silver Jubilee Medal and regret that I cannot personally pin this on you."

The parcel contained a sparkling siver medal about the size of a silver dollar and bearing the likeness of the King and Queen. There was also a certificate from Buckingham Palace, Coat of Arms and all, bear-

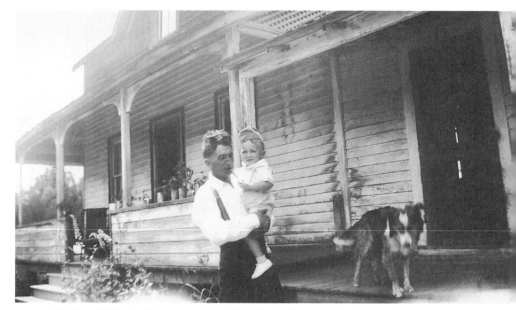

A'Delbert Miller holding young son, Melville, in front of their home in South Wilberforce. *Courtesy Virginia LeRoy Luckock Collection.*

ing these words: "By Command of HIS MAJESTY THE KING the accompanying Medal is forwarded to MISS GERTRUDE F. LEROY to be worn in commemoration of the Their Majesties' Silver Jubilee 6th May, 1935."

What an honour! I did not know what I had done to deserve such an award, but it is something to be mighty proud of.

By the next winter I had a little son[4] of my own so I was not available where nursing was concerned, at least for a little while. But before long, baby or not, I never knew when I might be called upon to help out. Nurses stayed at the Outpost only for short periods of time and I would be asked to fill in between postings. Sometimes women whom I'd attended previously would beg me to look after them, their reason being that they knew me and had confidence in me. But unless the nurse was away or the Outpost was without a nurse, I refused such cases. But whenever the nurse did go away, the stork seemed to pursue me as usual.

In March 1937, the nurse left very suddenly and I received an urgent request from Headquarters, asking me to please help out until they could get someone else. I could take my baby with me to the Outpost. Well, Del was at camp during the week (by this time I had learned to milk the cow) so he took the cow up to his father's. We closed our house, and I was back on the job, for six weeks.

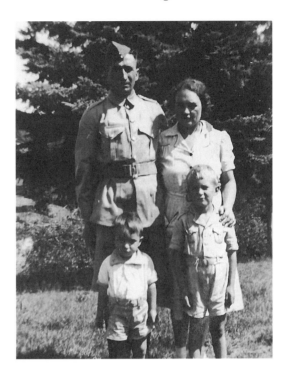

A family portrait. Del and Gertrude Miller with sons, Gerald Richard (known in area as Dick) and elder son Melville Charles. *Courtesy Virginia LeRoy Luckock Collection.*

As usual, I found plenty to do. By this time Aileen had left,[5] and the girl who was there was anything but a housekeeper in my opinion. But there was no one else available. I was worried when it was necessary to leave her to look after a patient while I was out on a call. I usually took my son to his grandmother's where he was always welcome.

Sometimes the Red Cross Committee put on a dance in February or March to relieve the monotony of the winter months, as well as raise a little money to help carry on. This year one had been planned for March 17th and, from all reports, a large crowd was expected. Several women had gathered at the Outpost during the afternoon to make suppertime sandwiches and other food. By food time the place was stacked with cakes and other goodies that had been brought in. The big boiler was on the stove filled with water for the tea and all the preparations were complete. We had a patient at the time, but her husband was coming to spend the evening with her, which greatly relieved my mind. I would be able to slip over to the hall once in a while for some fun.

The roads were good and by eight o'clock cars were beginning to arrive, as well as horses and cutters or sleighs, as well as many people on foot. About eight-thirty it started to snow a little, but we didn't think much about it. We had been so lucky so far, having little snow. Many had been using their cars all winter. Quite a crowd had gathered and the fiddlers were tuning up.

I was on my way back to the Outpost for something when a car drove up and stopped at the gate. The driver, Russell S. called to me, "Mrs. T. needs you right away," he said, "I told them I'd bring you."

I assured him I would be ready in a few minutes. In I went to change my clothes and make arrangements with the housekeeper regarding the patient and my son, in case I should be late returning.

It was an eight-mile drive and by the time we reached our destination it was snowing quite hard. This was the third time I had delivered this patient so she knew pretty well what preparations to make. She was a most co-operative person and always tried to have everything just right. There was not much for me to do except scrub up and get out my sterile things.

In about two hours everything was over. Mr. and Mrs. T. now had ten children. Finally, the baby was bathed and asleep, the mother comfortable and happy. The room was tidied and I was ready to leave.

By that time the snow was quite deep and still falling fast. However, Russell, who was still waiting for me, said he was quite sure we could make the trip all right. Mr. T. said he would come along and bring a shovel in case we did get stuck. Well, we might have got along fine if the road had been perfectly level, but it wasn't. Every dip was filled with snow. We had to be shovelled out four times in the first three miles, and by that time we had reached the Mumford home on top of a long hill, the height of land. From there we could not see the least sign of a road.

There was a light so we decided to go in to the house. I would either stay there until daylight, or perhaps their eldest son might take me on by horse and cutter. We all knew it was out of the question to get there by car.

Mrs. Mumford was up with the baby so invited us inside to get warm. She said that Eddie, their son, had gone to the dance with the horse and cutter and had not yet returned. However, if I would like to go on she was sure her husband would take me with the team and sleigh. By that time he was awake and came down and spoke for himself, saying he would be glad to take me. Since I was anxious to get back to my patient as well as my own child, I accepted his offer. The others started back with the car.

It was 4 a.m. when we reached the Outpost and, although there had been lots of straw and blankets on the sleigh, we were chilled right through. What a pleasure to find the kitchen nice and warm, and lots of sandwiches and cake that had been left from the dance. The kettle was simmering on the stove so it didn't take long to make some fresh coffee to fortify Mr. Mumford for his homeward journey.

The patient was awake and wondering what had happened to me. I made her comfortable and went to bed and to sleep, only to be awakened at seven-thirty by a loud thundering noise. It was a minute or two before I figured out that it was the big railroad snowplow going through.

After I had the patient and baby bathed and comfortable, and my other routine duties finished, the section foreman took me back to Harcourt on the gas car. It had taken us four hours to get home last night, but this time it took seven minutes to get to the crossing.

Now that era is over and forgotten. Many of the babies I helped into the world are now grandparents and remember nothing of the struggles of the Depression years, nor the joys and contentment that were experienced without all the luxury that these later years have provided and made us so important.

The Red Cross Outpost at Haliburton was finally realized in 1936. Then came the war, which brought about the development of many modern medicines and technologies which have changed the whole way of life.

Looking back, it was a wonderful experience for me. I derived more pleasure and satisfaction from my work as a Red Cross Nurse than I ever dreamed was possible. Always with a prayer in my heart for help and guidance from above, I knew no fear as I started out on my trips to the sick or tackled an emergency.

Incidently, everything was going according to the "THE PLAN." My dream of 1931 of expanding our Public Health program to include the whole of Haliburton County became a reality. In 1957, I was asked by the Ontario Department of Health and the County Council to take charge of that service, a position which I held for over ten years. When I retired, the Haliburton Kawartha Pine Ridge District Health Unit was formed.

I realize that the part I played was, on the whole, very small. I was just one person working in a very small area of our great Dominion of Canada. My only wish is that some people benefitted from my having been there to help in their time of need. There are many more doing the same and even more worthwhile work, but the need is still very great, especially among the Native Peoples of our country. How nice it would be to be young again!

Epilogue

Gertrude and A'Delbert Miller made their home permanently in Wilberforce in the "Cottage" Gertrude had purchased from Del's Uncle Joe and Aunt Mary Dunford. Sons Melville Charles and Gerald Richard were born to them. Del spent some of World War II in the Army. The boys rode the buses to public school in Wilberforce and high school in Haliburton Village. Throughout these years, in addition to all the duties of being mother and wife, Gertrude was involved in the local United Church and in other community work, often as the leader/organizer. Her creative talents were expressed in oil paintings, leather crafts, quilts and sewing. Some of her works were sold, many were given away to family and friends. She continued to assist at the Outpost when needed and gave competent leadership in the Wilberforce branch of the Red Cross.

The Red Cross ceased operation of the Wilberforce Outpost in 1957. Larger Hospitals were now accessible in neighbouring villages. The Corporation known as the Monmouth Charitable Association, (mainly the same people who formed the Wilberforce branch of the Ontario Division of the Canadian Red Cross) had owned the building on behalf

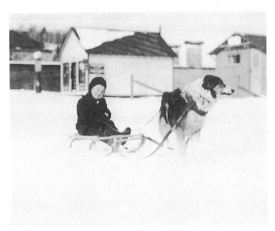

A young Melville Miller being pulled on a sleigh by his dog, along the main road through Wilberforce in the early 1940s. The main building visible to the left is Mrs. Shay's store and to the right, the Post Office (Frank Schofield, Postmaster), with a glimpse of the Veneer Factory in the distant background. *Courtesy The Virginia LeRoy Luckock Collection.*

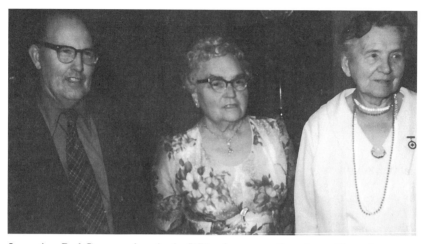

Long time Red Cross workers in the Wilberforce area. From l to r: Kenneth Sanderson, Gertrude LeRoy Miller and May Croft. Circa 1981. *Courtesy Ken and Nadeen Sanderson.*

of the community since the early 1920s. With public approval, the property was deeded to Monmouth Township in 1963 and was rented out as a private residence until 1989.

Just as the Red Cross Outpost service in Wilberforce was ending in the late 1950s, the Ontario Department of Health and Haliburton County Council asked Gertrude to take charge of a county wide Public Health Program. Bessie (Lee) Croft who worked as Gert's secretary for a number of years recalls Mrs. Miller as a very intelligent woman. Bessie respected her dedication to her work and deeply admired her creative abilities in painting and other crafts.

Hilda Clark, who grew up in the village, remembers Gertrude as a well-spoken woman who loved to lead, and was impressed that she, a woman, owned and drove her own car.

Sylvia (Battersby) Cameron recalled working with Gertrude and local nurses Marion (Campbell) Tallman and Ruth (Sanderson) Saunders when they presented a well-received Home Nursing Course in the community after the Outpost service ended. (Mrs. Sylvia Cameron[1] herself was a well respected Red Cross Outpost Nurse in Wilberforce in the late 1930s. After the Outpost closed, Sylvia worked out of her home for the Red Cross. Marion Tallman served at the Outpost in the fifties).

Kenneth Sanderson, a lifetime resident of Wilberforce, knew the author well. He worked with Gertrude in the work of the Wilberforce Branch of the Ontario Division of the Canadian Red Cross, and in the Wilberforce Home and School Association. He remembers her "as a very determined person, an individual who put the concerns of others ahead of her own, very compassionate for the less fortunate. For her there was no task too large, no goal too small."

Forty-three years after her "temporary" placement at the Outpost, Gertrude LeRoy Miller departed from the Wilberforce area. In 1974, widowed, her two sons now adults and living elsewhere in the province, Gertrude sold her home, the "Cottage," which she had acquired as a young nurse. For a brief period she lived in Peterborough, then moved to London, Ontario where she resided until her death on December 18, 1983.

The *Echo and Recorder*, a Haliburton County weekly, on Wednesday, January 11, 1984, published a report submitted after her death. "Gertrude F. Miller was a friend to countless people wherever she lived. Gertrude was an extremely talented woman. Her crafts were always beautifully executed, and her paintings grace many walls throughout the county.[2] Gertrudes's talent for organizing was another attribute and the Haliburton and District Association for the Mentally Retarded was one of her pet projects: she was a Charter Member.

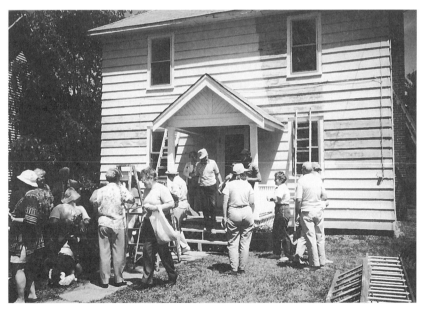

Once the decision was made to recognize the historical significance of the Red Cross Outpost, there was much to be done. A "neighbourhood party" (1992) pitching in to help restore the building in readiness for its new life. *Courtesy Hilda Clark.*

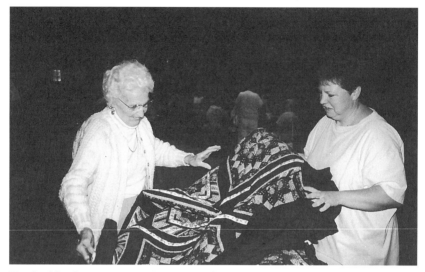

Fund raising became an ongoing priority for the Wilberforce Heritage Guild. Here, Cathy Agnew, right, the President, presents a handmade quilt to the raffle winner, Edith Daniels in 1997. *Courtesy Hilda Clark.*

Gertrude's Christian character held her in good stead throughout her life. She was a member of the South Wilberforce United Church and the U.C.W. Her home was always the setting for the Christmas party.

"Gertrude's red Volkswagon was seen all over the county, visiting schools, always with a cheery greeting. She never lost her zest for life.

"A memorial service was held in South Wilberforce United Church, December 28, 1983...her final act of an unselfish life was the donation of her body to science."

Meanwhile, the Outpost had been home to a number of families, being rented to them by Monmouth Township. It became vacant in 1989 and needed a saviour. A group of interested, concerned citizens, recognizing the building's historical importance as the *FIRST* Red Cross Outpost Hospital and its potential value, formed the Wilberforce Heritage Guild and began to take responsibility for it in March 1991.

With great community support, especially from Monmouth Township Council, and lots of volunteer labour, the Outpost reopened as an Historic House Museum on August 15, 1992. Almost half a century of one aspect of local history has been preserved and made available for public enjoyment and education. The "Outpost" once again serves the public in Monmouth and area.

Epilogue

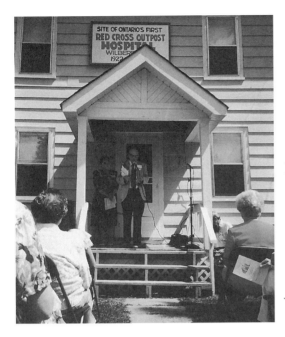

All the hard work is rewarded. On August 15, 1992, the Wilberforce Red Cross Outpost Museum is officially opened. Positioned on the platform, the newly refurbished porch entrance, are Cathy Agnew and Ken Sanderson. *Courtesy Wilberforce Heritage Guild.*

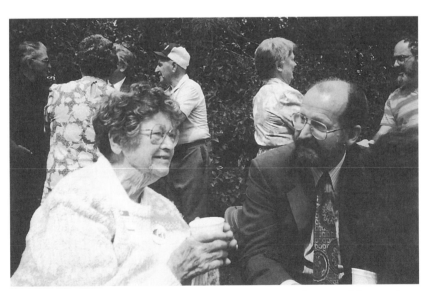

Previous Outpost Nurses and their families were invited to be part of the opening celebrations. Elizabeth (Daisy) Knaggs Lean, an Outpost nurse from 1925 to 1928, enjoys some refreshments with her son, David Lean. At the time she was 95 years of age. In the background are: Melville Miller; Flo Taylor (with her back to the camera); Keith Tallman; Jack Daniels and Doreen Croft Hutchinson talking to John Sloan, the United Church minister.

187

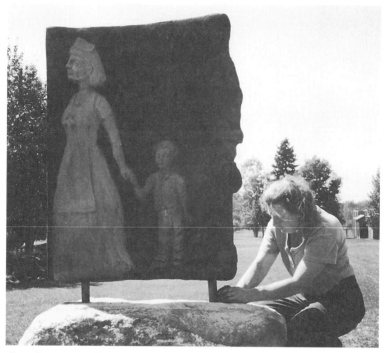

Jane Agnew puts finishing touches to her sculpture, honouring the nurses of the Wilberforce Red Cross Outpost Hospital. *Courtesy Hilda Clark.*

A sculpture depicting a young nurse, forward-looking and determined, with a firm yet gentle hand extended to a child, can be seen in the park as one enters Wilberforce. Created by North Bay area sculptor, Jane Agnew, a frequent instructor at the Haliburton School of Fine Arts, it was installed on September 3, 1999. This is one of a "Garden of Sculptures" placed in community parks throughout the county through the initiative of the Haliburton County Development Corporation's Art Committee.

This sculpture celebrates the contribution of the nurses who served the community from the Wilberforce Red Cross Outpost Hospital (1922–1963)–the *first* in Ontario. Gertrude LeRoy Miller, a nurse and an artist, would have approved.

Hilda G. J. Clark
Past President, Wilberforce Heritage Guild

Appendix A
Monmouth Charitable Association—1922–1963

The original members of the Corporation known as the Monmouth Charitable Association founded in 1922 to acquire the Red Cross Nursing Service were:

Gerald A. Finlay, Tory Hill

Frances D. Herlihey, Tory Hill

Herbert S. Mulloy, Wilberforce

Rev. Joseph W. Ogden, Wilberforce

Stanley W. Reynolds, Wilberforce

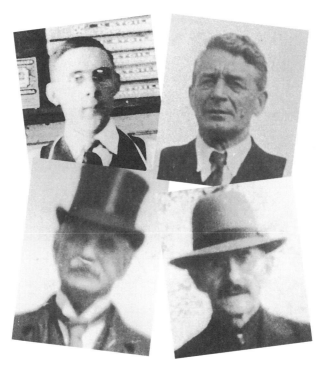

Clockwise from top left: Gerald A. Finlay, Frances D. Herlihey, Herbert S. Mulloy and Rev. Joseph W. Ogden. (No photograph of S. W. Reynolds available) *Courtesy Wilberforce Heritage Guild.*

Appendix B

Red Cross Nurses at Wilberforce—(1922–1957)

Red Cross Nurses known by the Wilberforce Heritage Guild to have served at the Wilberforce Red Cross Outpost Hospital. Married names, as known, are shown in brackets.

Josephine Jackson (Whebell)	February 1922–1923
Catherine Lawrence	October 1923–1924
Anne Casey	1924–1925
Elizabeth Knaggs (Lean)	1925–1928
Jean Marie Lougheed	1928–1929
Bessie Stirling (Wilson)	1929–1930
Gertrude F. LeRoy (Miller)	September 10, 1930–August 31, 1934
Miss G. Farrar	1935
Gladys Reid	1935–1936
Sylvia Battersby (Cameron)	1936–1938
I. Gardiner	1938
A. Whittaker	1939
S.I. Mogk	1939, 1941
Miss Gardner	1940
V. (Polly) Nelson	1941–1942
Victoria Rains (Agnew)	1943–1945
Elsie Turner (Metcalfe)	1946–1948
Miss Hyslop	1950
Helen Singer and Edith Chapman, who were also Eastern Ontario Supervisors of Red Cross Outpost Nurses, also spent some time in Wilberforce.	1950
Marion Campbell	December 1950–September 1952
Mrs. Dorie Kenny	1952–1957

Others that served during the 1950s for short periods: Louise Grover, Miss M. Chattoe, Eileen Warren, Evelyn Barry Edwards, Mary Whitmore (substitute nurse).

Student nurses: Miss Walker, student nurse during Gertrude LeRoy's time at Outpost. Ruth MacDonald and Jean Scrimgeur also known to have been student nurses.

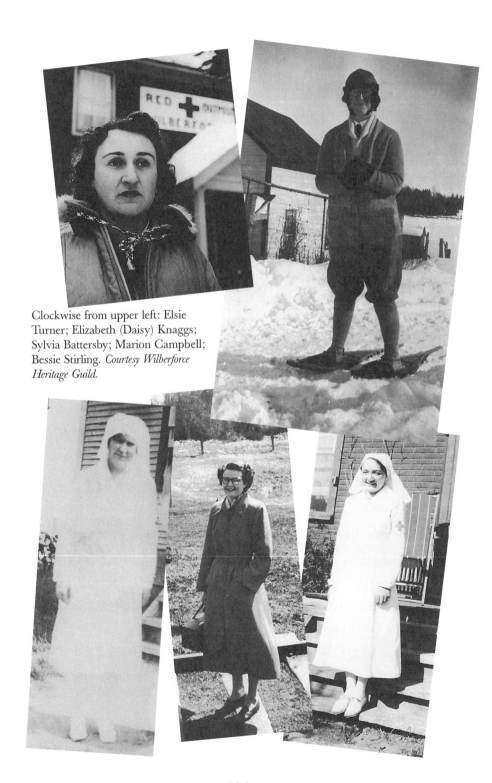

Clockwise from upper left: Elsie
Turner; Elizabeth (Daisy) Knaggs;
Sylvia Battersby; Marion Campbell;
Bessie Stirling. *Courtesy Wilberforce
Heritage Guild.*

Appendix C

Pupils Attending Local Schools in the early 1930s[1]

WILBERFORCE, JUNIOR ROOM
Teacher: Miss Margory Chambers–November, 1931

Elmer Sanderson
Edith Tallman
Isobel Fleming
Evelyn Rowe
Mary Coulthard
Wilbur Sanderson
Aileen Fleming
Kathleen Fleming
Madeline Bowen
Clifford Godfrey
Jimmie Miller
Harold Sequin
Helen Marshall

Doreen Croft
Clifford Fleming
Harry Clark
Royce Barnes
Jean Coulthard
Albert Sanderson
Leona Godfrey
Tommy Marshall
Murray Agnew
Ernie Tallman
Elmer Scott
Florence Sequin
Casey Marshall

Kenneth Sanderson
Iris Bowen
Ruth Rowe
Eddie Scott
Fred Wright
Eddie Ackley (Ted)
David Croft
Jean Tallman
George Wright
Jacqueline Sequin
Earle Mumford
Ronald Mumford

WILBERFORCE SENIOR ROOM
Teacher: Miss Elizabeth (Betty) Byers[2]–November, 1931

Irma Bowen
Isobel Coulthard
George Earle
Arthur Fleming

Stanley Fleming
Daisy Hillis
Robert Marshall
Lloyd Bowen

BEECH RIDGE–June, 1932

Bridget Elliott
Luella Elliott
Violet Milne
Lillie Milne

Tommy Elliott
Bessie Bowers
Billie Elliott
Dorothy Stoughton

Vernon Stoughton
Gordon Stoughton
Guy Farrel

HIGHLAND GROVE (Cardiff #4) (The North School)
Teacher: Miss Dorothy Switzer[3]–November, 1931

Mabel Hubble
Mary Hubble
Ferol Lewis
Warnie Peel
Asa Leedy
Loyal Bowen
Gerald Covert
Lavern Lewis
Wilda Hubble
Fay Sucie
Clifford Hubble
James Bamford

Morley Bowen
Carl Lewis
Eunice Bamford
Galen Covert
Leola Covert
Grace Lewis
Ormand Bamford
Lorne Sucie
Herman Lewis
Elsie Hubble
Elaine Bamford
Elmer Covert

Orland Lewis
Junior Bowen
Shirley Covert
May Leedy
Norma Covert
Jean Lewis
Helen Morgan
Olive Bamford
Jack Morgan
Joe Storey
Gordon Storey

HIGHLAND GROVE (Cardiff #3) (The South School)
Teacher: Mr. Roland Sedgwick[4]–1931

Stella Mitchell
Amy Foster
Annie Hughey
Ila Andrews
Elsie Bowen
Irwin Bowen
Winnifred Bowen
Violet Hogan
Everett Hogan

Vern Hughey
Jeanne Landry
Erma Watson
Evelyn Andrews
Tresa Hogan
Douglas Landry
Norman Bowen
Daisy Bowen
Marvin Bowen

Allen Foster
Jean Hogan
Garfield Hogan
Harry Hogan
Clem Hogan
Irene Hogan
Warren Bowen
Marvin Hughey
Eileen Bowen

ESSONVILLE
Teacher: Mrs. Julia Biggs[5]–September, 1931

Randall McCrea
Lorne Woolacott
Evie Payne
Hilden Johnston
Leonard Henry
Elda Henry
Alma Gibson
Russell Henry

Dorothy Rowbotham
Gladys Henry
Herbie Henry
Irene Johnston
Carl Sibley
Margaret Rowbotham
Nellie Somerville

Eddie Somerville
May Rowbotham
Jim Gibson
Russell Gibson
Florence Henry
Eldon Sibley
Sidney Henry

HARCOURT–1931

Harcourt Pacey
Violet Scott
Clayton Scott
Jean Scott
Etta Pacey
Betty Pacey

Gordon Scott
Hazel Townsend
Pearl Pacey
Bruce Scott
Lyman Townsend

Elsworth Scott
Elwood Townsend
Murray Scott
Wallace Scott
Wesley Scott

KENNAWAY
Teacher: Miss Hazel Miller–October, 1931

Eleanor Palmateer	Myrtle Holbrook	Milton Cox
Russell Holbrook	Wilfred Holbrook	Bernard Palmateer
Jane Palmateer	Bernice Cox	Violet Holbrook

CHEDDAR
Teacher: Mrs. Annie Nesbitt[6]–September, 1931

Donald McGregor	Howard Baumhauer	Teenie Evans
Phyllis Jeffrey	Teddie Evans	Elsie Evans
Willie Baumhauer	Cassie Evans	Roy Bates
Lela McGregor	Elsie Bates	Max Peters
Florence Jeffrey	Jack Jeffrey	Marie Peters
Bessie Evans	Bessie Bates	Hazel Sweet
Gladys Bates	May Sweet	Leonard Evans

TORY HILL
Teacher: Miss Margaret Hanthorne[7]–1932

Ira Bowen	Joe Day	Lorene Dack
Douglas Atherley	Helen Atherley	Vivian Gill
Audrey Bonham	Mary Dack	Elwin Short
Ruby Johnson	Roy Gibson	Lillie Maguire
Jim Dack	Madeline Lee	Loral Coumbs
Stephen McCrea	Gerald Johnson	Lois Atherley
Willie Boyce	Norman Lee	Madeline Dack
Ross Anderson	Alberta Gibson	Vera Gill
Florence Maguire		

Notes

All endnotes have been developed by Hilda Clark, based on her general knowledge of the area, except for those identified as having a specified source.

1 NOT A STRANGER FOR LONG

1 Gertrude did eventually sketch and paint this landscape. Some of her artworks have been included in this book.
2 According to her sister Virginia LeRoy Luckock, Gertrude had hoped to be a missionary. She apparently expected to be sent further afield than Wilberforce to apply her missionary goal to nursing.
3 According to Wilberforce Heritage Guild records, the nurse she replaced was Elizabeth (Bess) Stirling.
4 Records at the Outpost Historic House indicate that a very attractive verandah across the front of the house was lost when the whole building was moved back from the street and placed on a new basement. Lack of funds and plenty of lumber resulted in the "ugly" new porch.
5 Aileen Ames eventually married Fred Walker of Brooks, Alberta. At time of publication Aileen is widowed and retired in Edmonton. She keeps in touch with friends and family in Ontario. Many pictures on display at the Outpost were donated by Aileen.
6 The Outpost and most frame houses at that time were sheeted inside and out with lumber which was plentiful in the area. Cracks were covered by pasting on cloth or paper, then wallpapered.
7 Local sources suggest that they were Lorne Marshall and Earle Fleming.
8 According to a letter, dated February 10, 1930 from Miss Ruby Hamilton, Nursing Supervisor, to Miss Bess Stirling R.N., the gyproc was donated by Canada Gypsum and Alabastine Ltd. of Brantford, Ontario. A Mr. Wilson of that company informed the Ontario Division of the Canadian Red Cross of the donation by letter.
9 The toilet, also called outhouse or backhouse.
10 St. Margaret's Anglican Church established in 1920. There had been an Anglican presence in the area for many years. Christ Church, Essonville, was established in 1888. Originally, St. Margaret's Church was a bunk house owned by the Spears and Lauder Lumber Company. It was moved from its original location across the street from Agnew's General Store by John Holmes, using log rollers with horses to tow it to its present site a few hundred metres to the north.

The building was renovated and church windows added. Pews from the Cheddar Anglican Church, which had been closed, were brought in as furnishings.

11 The first school in the Wilberforce area, a wooden frame building, was built in 1893 near the Methodist (later United) Church. It was situated across from the cemetery in what is now referred to as South Wilberforce (actually the original Wilberforce settlement). Later, about 1900, as more people settled in what is presently the village of Wilberforce, another school was established where the Terrace Inn now stands. In 1911, this structure was replaced by a new brick building, also a one-room school. With a growing enrolment and the need for higher education, another room and a large hallway were added in 1921. This expanded building was the Consolidated Continuation School, known as S.S. 6 & 8 Cardiff and Monmouth, located in Wilberforce that Gertrude LeRoy was shown on her first evening at the Outpost.

Over the years, classes have varied from Grades 1 to 13 in the early 1940s to Kindergarten to Grade 4 in the late 1980s early 1990s, ultimately becoming Junior Kindergarten to Grade 6 in 2000.

12 Aileen was not far from her home. Her father, Ezrom Ames, and stepmother, Tamar, lived just across the street. Her mother, Alice (Graham) Ames, was deceased. Her aunt, Isabel (Graham) Shay, lived next door to the Outpost.

13 The train that Gertrude took to Wilberforce and used a great deal. It was the Irondale, Bancroft, and Ottawa Railway operating between Bancroft and Howland Junction (near Kinmount). It made stops in Irondale, Gooderham, Tory Hill, Wilberforce, Harcourt, Highland Grove and Baptiste. The railway had many nicknames, including "the I.B.& Slow."

14 This would have been Fred Agnew.

15 Flora (Webber) Marshall. Their stone house was later sold to Harold and Beatrice (Schickler) Herlihey. At time of publication, Beatrice, widowed, is not in the best of health.

16 Bertha Webber, daughter of Jane and George Webber.

17 The children of Charles and Viva Bowen were Elgin, Irma, Lloyd, Madeline and Iris.

18 George and Melissa (Dunford) Miller's children were Mary, A'Delbert, Hazel, George (Geordie) and James (Jimmy).

19 This was Bertha (Clark) Minns White.

20. Bertha White's mother was Mary Anne (Graham) Clark

21 Miss Annie Taylor, an Anglican Deaconess who ministered from St. Margaret's Anglican Church, lived at the local boarding house.

22 Operated by the Loyal Orange Order, this was the community hall. It was torn down in 1971, and the Monmouth Library was built on the site.

23 The same trip in 2000 would take about twenty-five minutes!

24 Louisa Earle, widow of William Earle, eventually had a new frame house built across the road in 1933, where she lived well into her nineties. At time of publication, George Earle, her son, still resides in the house. The log house shown on the back cover is a painting of the Earle's log house. It was painted by Gertrude Miller, framed by the Wilberforce United Church Women (U.C.W.) and given to Mrs. Earle on her 90th birthday.

25 Hilda Clark recalls how special it was to have Mrs. Earle visit. "If we youngsters

were polite and asked nicely and listened well, she would tell our fortunes by reading tea leaves in our cups at the end of the meal. We noticed that our father (Walter) always swished his tea leaves around and drank them so his cup couldn't be read!"

2 MEET THE CHALLENGE: HIT THE FLOOR RUNNING

1 According to documents held by the Wilberforce Heritage Guild, both Bess Stirling, the "departing nurse," and Gertrude LeRoy attended a meeting of the Wilberforce Red Cross Branch (Committee) at the Outpost on September 29, 1930. The minutes of the meeting record: " that Miss Stirling proposed, seconded by Mrs. F. (Clara) Schofield that Ruth Sanderson and Grace Saunders be added to the R. Committee. Motion carried." It would appear that the departing nurse had stayed in the area, perhaps with friends, to attend the September 29th meeting. If this was the meeting that the author describes later in this chapter, it is interesting that she makes no mention of Miss Stirling attending.

2 It appears that Gertrude's first maternity case was Elizabeth (Lizzie), wife of Robert Elliott.

3 This "Maternity Kit" was a large black leather suitcase with specially designed cloth pockets lining its sides, designed to hold the necessary bottles, brushes and other small items. A large Red Cross in a white circle was painted on the lid.

4 The Victorian Order of Nurses (V.O.N.) founded in 1898, "despite fierce opposition from the medical establishment" *Canadian Encyclopedia* page 2-3, by Lady Ishbel Aberdeen, wife of the Governor-General of Canada (1893–1898), is still in operation.

5 Kathleen (Mrs. John Stapley) was born September 14, 1930. Kay confirms that Gertrude LeRoy delivered her. The uncle with the bad brakes was likely John Schickler.

6 See Chapter Six for information on the part played by the Monmouth Charitable Association in getting the Red Cross Outpost Service established in Wilberforce.

7 From 1922 to 1930, about 60 babies had been born in Monmouth Township.

8 Though the Outpost building no longer relies on a hand pump, the water system occasionally still causes problems for the Heritage Guild at the museum!

3 DEALING WITH LONELINESS

1 Gertrude took her training for nursing at Toronto Western Hospital.

2 Aileen Ames' father Ezrom, a well-remembered violin player, and his second wife Tamar, who played piano, were likely two of the musicians, the "dance committee" obtained to play for the dance.

3 This may have been Leonard Holmes. A picture of him on page 48 of Richard Pope's book *Me 'n Len* (Dundurn Press 1985) shows him to have been "tall, dark and handsome" and he certainly was still a bachelor in 1930. Another Leonard living in Wilberforce at that time was Leonard Fleming. He, being a fiddler, was more likely to have been one of the musicians for the dance!

4 Handcar, as used in the title of this book is a general term used to describe several different kinds of small rail vehicles used by railroad workers. These handcars were used to transport themselves, their tools and other materials to inspect,

maintain and repair their section of the railway. Knowledgeable, former railway employees, such as Geroge Grant of Wilberforce and Victor Snider of Gooderham, have confirmed this information. The Webster's Dictionary also confirms this description with the following definition: "Handcar–a small four-wheeled railroad car propelled by a hand-operated mechanism or by a small motor."

Often Gertrude LeRoy was able to have the section foreman or one of his crew transport her on such a handcar, enabling her to reach people in need of medical assistance. She often refers to the handcar as a gas car because it was powered by a one-cylinder motor. This gas car was a great advancement over earlier models. These vehicles were light enough to be lifted on and off the rails by hand. Many handcars were made by the Sylvester Company in Lindsay, Ontario.

5 Cheddar, once a thriving community is now a ghost town. According to Mrs. Elsie (Bates) Earle, who attended the Cheddar School, it was a frame building painted red, hence the name Red School was commonly used. Later, she became the school caretaker, and remembers how difficult it was to keep the school heated in winter.

6 Mrs. Elsie (Bates) Earle, one of Mrs. Nesbitt's former students, remembered her well and provided her first name. She recalls Mrs. Nesbitt taking her (Elsie) and her cousin Gladys Bates (who later married Bill Ponkhazi) home for a few days. This was, interestingly, at a place called Elsie, a settlement between Minden and Carnarvon, Ontario. Mrs. Earle, whose late husband Stephen was one of the sons of the teacup reader Louisa Earle (Chapter 1), recalls Gertrude LeRoy giving herself and some other students who were walking, a ride to school in her car.

7 Little remains of the Hotspur settlement which was in the southwestern-most part of Monmouth Township. That area began to be settled when, in 1871, the Monck Road, which ran from Lake Simcoe to the Hastings County boundary, passed through South Monmouth. According to the book, *Monmouth Township 1881–1981, Collected Views of the Past* (1981), the original settlers' school was replaced: "The new frame school was built around 1900 and is still standing [1981] and is used as a summer home. Inside the interior is covered with beautifully scrolled metallic walls, as was the fashion at the turn of the century. It was not until 1920 that yearly school was held." This would have been the school Gertrude LeRoy visited in the early 1930s.

8 Junior Red Cross was an organization found in many schools. Students formed an executive and held meetings/programs on occasional Friday afternoons to raise awareness of a healthy life style. Pins and health rule cards were given to all students each year. As well, the program provided leadership opportunities.

9 This was the home of Merle (Cornell) and Clifford Avey. The little girls, victims of the fire, were Fern, age 7, and June, age 5. The fire took place in November of 1930. Information was confirmed by Ethel (Avey) Smith, sister of the fire victims.

4 BOOKS BRING PRINCE CHARMING
AND OTHER CHARMING CUSTOMS

1 "Calling" was the singing out of the step instructions for the square dances.
2 Murray Agnew of Agnew's General Store, a lifelong Wilberforce resident and postmaster, well remembers seeing George Miller, Del's father, carry this velocipede home. He would take it from the point where the I.B.&O. Railway crossed

the Burleigh Road, now Haliburton County Road 648, and along the main street through the village. Mr. Miller simply took the "pede" apart and carried it over his shoulder, passing Agnew's as he went.

3 These catalogues would have been from the T. Eaton Co. (ceased to exist in 1999), and the Robert Simpson Co., now the Hudson Bay Company.

4 Doris Schofield, often called Doll, married George Wells of Cambray. Widowed, she later married Dr. Stewart Wilson, a dentist in the Lindsay area..

5 GETTING THERE IN WINTER IS HALF THE TASK

1 Gertrude LeRoy is likely referring to the time of her writing of this manuscript, believed to have been in the late 1960s and early 1970s.

2 In the text, Gertrude refers to the handcar, a small four-wheeled railway vehicle she often used, as the gas car.

3 From notes submitted by Virginia LeRoy Luckock to Hilda Clark: Charles Lafayette LeRoy (1874–1965) blacksmith and Emma Frances LeRoy (1879–1945) dressmaker, were born in Ontario and lived near Chatham and Alvinston, Ontario. They moved to Detroit, Michigan, where Charles worked for R.E. Olds (maker of the Oldsmobile) in a shop located across the road from Henry Ford. Charles and his brothers, Fred and Frank, helped build the car called "The Northern." Charles was the first man to put a steering wheel and a gearshift on a car. Eventually he made a career shift and went into the grocery business.

When they moved back to Canada in July 1918 with the four children, Charles stayed in the grocery business for several years. The children: Gertrude Frances LeRoy b. February 10, 1902 d. December 18, 1983; Reta Lilas LeRoy (Keay) b. June 15, 1905 d. April 2, 1986; Donald James LeRoy b. March 5, 1913 d. November 1, 1985; Emma Virginia LeRoy (Luckock) b. September 26, 1915. Later, Charles took up the ornamental iron business until he retired. Emma Frances was a stay-at-home mom and a good friend to all.

6 ENTERPRISING VILLAGE GETS FIRST
ONTARIO RED CROSS OUTPOST HOSPITAL

1 One of the physicians was Dr. Herbert Walker, who lived in the house between the Wilberforce School and the Anglican Church.

2 Burleigh Road was a north/south colonization road.

3 Kenneth Sanderson believes that Poverty Lake was officially renamed Wilbermere Lake in the early 1920s at the request of the Sanderson family, who operated Wilbermere Farm, a tourist resort on its shores for several decades. It took many years for residents to call it by its new and more "positive" name.

4 Mrs. H.P. [Adelaide] Plumptre was the President of the Ontario Division of the Canadian Red Cross Society, the headquarters of which was in Toronto. She was still on the executive of that organization when Gertrude LeRoy was nurse-in-charge of the Wilberforce Outpost.

5 See Appendix A for list of nurses that the Wilberforce Heritage Guild's records show as having worked there.

6 As well as the Monmouth Charitable Association, a Corporation which, on behalf of the community, purchased and was *legally* responsible for the operation

of the Outpost, there was a Wilberforce Branch of the Ontario Division of the Canadian Red Cross, also referred to as the Committee, that was established in Wilberforce also in the early 1920s. Its first President was Eva (Mrs. George) Barnes and the secretary was Sophia (Mrs. Edward) Sanderson. Records show that many of the same people served on both the Corporation and the Red Cross Branch or Committee. They all worked very vigorously to keep the Nursing Service at the Outpost.

7 The author's opinion,concerning the reasons for the short stays of some of the nurses that preceded her, was not shared by all residents that were helped by them.

8 See Appendix C for list of school children and their teachers in the early 1930s.

9 The Imperial Order of Daughters of the Empire (I.O.D.E.) was founded in 1900 by Margaret Polson Murray of Montreal, to promote "things British" through the schools. Many branches of I.O.D.E. were formed across Canada.

7 WHEELS MAKE A DIFFERENCE

1 This was known as the Maternity Kit. It is a valued artifact presently on display at the Outpost Historic House in Wilberforce, Ontario.

2 The notes of Dr. J. Bruce Frain of Winnipeg, concerning his father, concur greatly with the author's stories. For example, he writes: " He [Dr, Charles E. Frain] delivered babies, often with the help of local women, experienced in such matters (not formal midwives).Except in Wilberforce, babies were delivered at home and called for sometimes prolonged home visits in all weather. Wilberforce at that time had a Red Cross Hospital staffed by trained nurses, but no doctor in that village. This was also a convenient site for tonsillectomies."

3 Nurse [Elizabeth] Bess Stirling

4 Olean is a town in Cattahaugus County in New York State, U.S.A., about 75 miles south of Buffalo, near the Pennsylvania border.

5 Red Cross tags were small pieces of tagboard bearing the Red Cross symbol. These were tied with a string to a button or button hole to show that the bearer supported the cause. These were likely forerunners to the tag days, (apple days, daffodil days...) now held by many other organizations.

6 Donald LeRoy

7 Emma Frances LeRoy

8 POVERTY AND THE DEEPENING DEPRESSION

1 Miss Ruby E. Hamilton, Registered Nurse was the Nursing Supervisor for the Ontario Division of the Canadian Red Cross Society. Though she was in Toronto, she was actually Miss Gertrude LeRoy's supervisor or "boss." Gertrude had met her and Miss Maude Wilkinson, Assistant Director at the Red Cross Headquarters, while she (Gertrude) was taking her Public Health Nurse training after having received her R.N. It appears that it was Miss Hamilton who had suggested Miss LeRoy for the position at the Wilberforce Outpost.

2 Dr. S.S. Lumb was a Bancroft doctor.

3 Kennaway, a former settlement in Harcourt Township near Little Fishtail Lake, is sometimes spelled Kenneway.

Notes

9 INGENUITY KEEPS THE WOLF FROM MOST DOORS

1 Another sawmill was constructed in the village not many years later, only to be replaced in the 1940s by a factory that produced wood veneer instead of lumber. This factory, still operating at time of publication, employs about 35 people.
2 At night, beside the really steep logging roads, the men would dig a hole in the snowbank, build a fire and cover it tightly with large sticks of wood. Sand would be spread on top. In the morning, this hot sand would be mixed with coals from the fire. This mixture would be spread on the road so that the sleigh loads of logs with no brakes would slow down and not slide into the teams of horses pulling them.
3 A 1930's account book at the Outpost Museum indicates that supplying, sawing and splitting firewood for the Outpost furnance was a major effort each year. Suppliers and workers were often paid for the wood and/or labour.
4 Highway 35 passes through the Minden area in Haliburton County.

10 RECOLLECTIONS FROM A WATCHFUL NEIGHBOUR

1 Isabel Graham Shay's mother, Jane Clark, married William Graham. Jane's brother James Clark was married to William Graham's sister, Mary Anne. Jane, James and their mother, Margaret (Ferris) Clark, all fell victim to influenza/pneumonia and died within a month in 1890. Mary Anne simply moved her family in with her brother William, her bachelor brother Thomas Graham and their mother, Ellen (Kirkpatrick) Graham. Both families were raised together. (From the records of Hilda Clark).
2 This would be the Wilberforce United Church.
3 May (Mrs. Wilfred) Croft, at the time the book was being written, was widowed and had a home beside and just north of the United Church, across the road from the Wilberforce cemetery. Mrs. Croft, a well-known supporter of the Red Cross and a niece of Alfred and Frank Schofield, eventually moved into the village and lived there well into her 103rd year. She died February 15, 1992.
4 The Burleigh was a north-south colonization road.
5 At the end of Senior Fourth, or Grade 8, students wrote a test prepared by the Provincial Department of Education to gain "entrance" into High School.
6 The sisters (Isabel and Ella) boarded in Minden with their Aunt Alice (Clark) and Uncle Donald Hartle who kept a store there.
7 Her sister was Ella Graham who later married Daniel Neville.
8 Mrs. Shay may have been wrong about Fred Perry being a Bernardo boy.
9 Jim Mackness' daughter Elsie married Lloyd Watson, long-time Monmouth Township Clerk, after whom the Community Centre in Wilberforce is named.
10 This would be Thomas Graham.
11 Fred and Florence Perry later moved to Wilberforce to property overlooking Wilbermere Lake. Their son Hugh (nicknamed Bud) was the first baby born at the Wilberforce Red Cross Outpost Hospital. Their other children were Marguerite, Kathleen, Evelyn and Joan.
12 This school was where Terrace Inn (with cottages) is still located in 2000.
13 Beech Ridge School was between Harcourt and Wilberforce, on what today is known as the Mumford Road.

14 Mrs. Henry Pacey, was Ada Schickler, sister of Russell, and mother of Harcourt (Sonny), Etta, Pearl, Betty and George. In fact, George Pacey may have been the last, or one of the last babies to be born at the Outpost in Wilberforce.

15 George Earle was the brother-in-law to Louisa (Mrs. William Earle). George and his wife eventually moved to Haliburton Village where they established a store and their home at the corner of Highland Street and Hwy 118, where Black's Home Hardware is located (2000). It has been suggested that this George Earle was the first to own and drive a car in Wilberforce.

16 Ethel Hughey married Percy Paull, a Haliburton resident, who had moved west. They farmed at Coronation, Alberta. She died at age 109 in 1989.

17 Mable Hughey (1893–1983) married Walter Clark (1985–1970), and they were the parents of Bill (1916–1934), Edith (1918–1926), Harry (1922–1995), Elaine (1928–1990), Gordon and Hilda. Bill died in November 1934 in a Lindsay hospital. A leg broken in a horse and wagon accident was put in a cast at the Wilberforce Outpost. Three train days later (one week) a very ill person, he was taken to Lindsay. He died of gangrene. Edith died at the Outpost. She had been operated on for appendicitis there. Elaine, Gordon and Hilda were born at the Outpost.

18 Near where Isabel lived as a youngster, a hardwood bush was being cut down for cordwood. This wood was sent by rail to the village of Donald (near Minden, Ontario) to be processed into wood alcohol, acetates and charcoal at a huge chemical plant. (It is said that in 1908 this plant used 50 cords of wood a day.) Hence, the local people called this the Chemical Bush.

19 This crew of strangers were Italian immigrants who had been brought in to cut the cordwood. They would have been a new experience for young Isabel - different language, different foods! Timber cutting took a lot of "manpower." Since all logs had to be cut by hand with crosscut saws, into 48 inch lengths and then split. The story of these and other Italian families is well told in a small book entitled *They Worked and Prayed Together, the Italians of Haliburton County* (1988) by Leopolda z L. Dobrzensky. Many of the descendants of these hardworking, skilled, enterprising families still live and work and play in our county of Haliburton.

20 Aunt Annie was Mary Anne Graham (Mrs. James Clark) who had helped raise Isabel.

21 Ally was Isabel's older sister, Alice. Bertha Clark was her cousin. They all grew up in the same home. Ally married Ezrom Ames and they had three children: Phyllis (Mrs. Alf Willows, then Mrs. Olaf Abelson); Aileen (Mrs. Fred Walker) and Reginald.

22 Margaret Ritchie was the daughter of Robert and Elizabeth Ritchie.

23 Eva Croft married George Barnes. She had great leadership skills. A very able President of the Wilberforce Branch of the Red Cross, she worked extremely well for the cause for many years. Their family included Raymond, Lloyd and Blake. Though she had a crippled foot and wore a special shoe, she did not let this stop her from being a very active person.

24 This would be Walton Hughey who died of pneumonia at age 17 on March 17, 1912.

25 Mrs. Shay is referring to Mrs. Miller's brother, Donald LeRoy, who had purchased the Hillis property south of the cemetery.

26 Here she is referring to Mr. Wilson Earle. He and his wife Emma lived across the highway from the present (2000) public beach on Wilbermere Lake.

27 Mrs. Shay's name, Isabel, was often shortened to Belle, or Bebe.

28 The school was just north of the United Church. The Grahams, Holmes and Stevensons lived on part of the Haliburton Road now called Otter Lake Road. The Rileys lived just up the hill from where Otter Lake Road meets Hwy 648.

29 Flossie was likely Florence (Flossie) Holmes, sister of Ethel mentioned in this sentence. They lived near Isabel.

30 Lylah (probably should be spelled Lila) was Lila Stephenson, sister of Blanche mentioned in next sentence. They and their sister Muriel were daughters of Mr. & Mrs. George (Geordie) Stephenson. They also lived on the road Isabel Graham would have taken to church and school. Blanche Stephenson married Reg Givens, a top executive with the Ford Motor Company in Detroit, Michigan. Lila married George Taylor. Muriel married Stanley McCrae.

31 This was Jane (Clark) Graham.

32 Uncle Jim would be James Clark.

11   NO ROUTINE BECOMES ROUTINE

1 Wilfred Croft married May Schofield Barker, a niece of Frank and Alfred Schofield. Widowed, with son Herbert, May had emigrated from England to be with her uncles in Wilberforce. Story has it that she met Wilfred, a resident of Wilberforce, on the train between Montreal and Toronto when he was returning home from World War I. They met again in Wilberforce and were married. Their children were Doreen, David and Melville. Doreen, (Mrs. Aleck Hutchinson), was born at home in April 1922 with nurse Josephine Jackson in attendance and was the first baby born under the "new" Red Cross Outpost service. The Croft home at that time was about 6 miles from the Outpost in the south part of Wilberforce.

2 Edward Mumford is the eldest son of Arthur and Annie (Drumm) Mumford. At the time of publication (2000), he and his wife Mary live in Harcourt.

3 Likely Dr. Frain would not have been amused with this news because, according to Dr. J. Bruce Frain, his father Dr. Charles Frain, "...was a Baptist and believed in the Temperance Movement. I (Bruce) have been given to understand he helped the police in one or two raids on the local bootlegger."

12   AS NURSE'S ROLE EXPANDS, FAMILIES DO TOO

1 This appears to have been Mabel (Barnes) McIntyre, wife of Ken, whose first child, Joan, was born at the Wilberforce Outpost in March 1932, and second daughter Barbara, born there in 1933.

2 The woman may have been worrying about the higher cost of having a doctor. It was the time of tlhe Depression and many people were very short of cash.

3 Aileen (Ames) Walker sent pages from an autograph book she kept to the Wilberforce Guild. In it were autographs from three of these European students.

13   MIDWIVES, MODERN METHODS AND HOME REMEDIES

1 Hilda Clark recalls her Aunt Bertha White (as her mother Annie Clark had taught

her) making this salve from her "secret recipe." A few drops of carbolic acid, a disinfectant used in Carbolic Soap, was one ingredient. We called it horseshit salve. It really did heal! As long as Aunt Bertha was able to make it, there was always a jar at our house. Likely the disinfectant and the boiling of the manure killed any germs. At any rate, this salve healed many burns.

2 Quinsy as defined in a dictionary, is a severe inflammation of the throat or adjacent parts; it may include swelling and fever.

3 Maybe this is similar to cough medicines such as Buckley's Mixture!

4 You were to tie a used or soiled sock or stocking around your neck overnight! The warmth of it felt good after Mother had rubbed on the Rawleigh's Medicated Salve.

14   THE COTTAGE AND A TALE OF SCOUTS

1 Del's grandfather was Richard Dunford.

2 This would be Joseph Dunford.

3 Apparently, the sawmill was built by the previous owner, Isaac Ritchie, from whom Richard Dunford bought the place.

4 This area was the *original* Wilberforce, surrounded by farms, of course. The Methodist (now United) Church, the school, cemetery, cheese factory, the sawmill and the post office were all near Poverty (now Wilbermere) Lake and south of it on the Irondale River. (It was always known as Burnt River, but now people insist that this branch of the Burnt River is the Irondale River!) Two bridges spanned the river near the house that Gertrude LeRoy purchased as a "cottage." Eventually, it became her permanent home. As Gertrude suggests, the I.B.&O. railway was built to the north, and gradually the village shifted north as well.

5 According to the copy of deed provided by author's family, the property cost five hundred and seventy-five dollars ($575.00). The signing of deed was witnessed by Mary E. Agnew and F. G. Agnew.

6 Her brother-in-law, Stewart Keay was married to the author's sister, Reta. He was nicknamed "Cap" and appears to have been one of the scout leaders.

7 Stewart and Reta Keay.

8 This was the Orange Hall, which had a stage and roll-up curtain. It was the main spot for social activities.

9 This account of the camping trip of some of the Thirteenth Toronto Troop of Boy Scouts has been left as written in 1933 for their Scout bulletin.

15   PUTTING DOWN ROOTS WHILE MOVING ON

1 The solitaire was her engagement ring.

2 According to information received from Dr. Bruce Frain of Winnipeg, his father, Dr. Charles Frain, was not a strong swimmer. Apparently, he went swimming alone and drowned.

3 This is a strong reference to Del's parents.

4 Melville Charles. A second son Gerald Richard was born a few years later.

5 Aileen Ames had gone by train to visit her sister, Phyllis (Mrs. Alf Willows), in Brooks, Alberta. There she met and married Fred Walker. It would be many years later that she would return to Wilberforce for visits.

Notes

EPILOGUE

1 Sylvia Cameron died on Monday, January 24, 2000 in her eighty-ninth year, a greatly honoured citizen who will be long remembered for her exceptional service as a nurse and her dedication to her church, St. Margaret's, a loving mother, grandmother and great-grandmother.

2 The reference is to Haliburton County.

APPENDIX C

1 The student lists appear to be arranged in order of age, with the older students first and the younger ones at the end of each list

2 Elizabeth (Betty) Byers married Robert Herlihey of Tory Hill. He too was a school teacher. At this time (2000) Betty lives in Minden.

3 Elaine (Bamford) Holland provided us with her teacher's (Miss Switzer) first name which was Dorothy. Dorothy Switzer married Ken Lewis and they lived for many years on Baptiste Lake. Elaine well remembers that Miss Switzer was a strict disciplinarian!

4 Mr. Roland Sedgwick died in the mid-1990s as did his wife Edith (Edie), also a former teacher. They had lived in the Minden area for many years.

5 Reliable sources, Mrs. Gladys (Henry) McNeely of Wilberforce and Mrs. Nellie (Somerville) Strong of Essonville, clarified that their former teacher was Mrs. Biggs, not Briggs. Mrs. Nellie (Somerville) Strong believes her first name was Julia. She also recalls Gertrude LeRoy's much enjoyed visits to the school. Prizes were offered by Gertrude for the best "Health" project in words and pictures. Nellie was delighted to have her project judged the best of the girls' work. She won a doll. Evie Payne, also at Nellie's school, won a ball for the boy with the best project.

6 Mrs. Elsie (Bates) Earle remembered that Mrs. Nesbitt's first name was Annie.

7 Madeline (Lee) Halek kindly provided her teacher Miss Margaret Hanthorne's first name.

Acknowledgements

The Wilberforce Heritage Guild accepted the challenge of bringing about the publishing of this book, a long standing goal expressed by the late Gertrude LeRoy Miller. This publication is viewed as part of the work of preserving and promoting the history of Wilberforce and area. The dedication of the members and Board of Directors of the Wilberforce Heritage Guild is much appreciated.

Thank you to Gertrude Miller's sons and heirs, Melville Charles Miller and Gerald Richard Miller for their permission to publish this edition of the book. Thanks are also due to the Municipality of Monmouth for its confidence and generous financial assistance on behalf of its residents. In addition, both the financial support of the Community Economic Development Committee of the Haliburton County Development Corporation and their confidence in the project are deeply appreciated. Indeed, the Wilberforce Heritage Guild is indebted to all the people who have wholeheartedly supported our many and varied fund raising activities for the book.

We are grateful to Virginia LeRoy Luckock, sister of the author, and to Gloria Luckock Wigg, niece, for their consistent support and encouragement. To Tracey Nottage for the initial work on the Index, the proofreading and the getting of the manuscript on computer disk so efficiently, we give a big thanks.

The wonderful help given by so many people to ensure correct information, particularly names, for the Notes and the Index and the visuals is greatly valued.

With appreciation, the Wilberforce Heritage Guild recognizes the following for their financial contributions: Murray & Eileen Agnew; Ross & Victoria Agnew; Barbara Weir & Joan Chubb; Hilda G.J. Clark; Gary & Patricia Collins; Bessie & Melville Croft; Jayne Elliott; Donna, Jim, Kira, and Kyle Fry; Margaret Harrison; Doreen (Croft) Hutchinson; Kemcroft Enterprises; Cathy LeRoy, Susan & Alex LeRoy; Elsie Lewis; Virginia (LeRoy) Luckock; Diane (Didi) Miller; Melville & Jeanna Miller; Sue Newell; Alfretta O'Rourke; Steve & Marlene Robertson; Kathy & Stephen Rogers; Wendell & Lorna (Keay) Sedgwick; Fred & Florence Taylor; Aileen Ames Walker; Wilberforce Ladies Auxiliary Branch 624 of the Royal Canadian Legion.

Other Books of Interest

Leopolda z L. Dobrzensky. *Fragments of a Dream*. Municipality of Dysart et al: 1985

Leopolda z L. Dobrzensky, *They Worked and Prayed Together: Italians in Haliburton County*. Haliburton, Ontario: 1988.

Monmouth Township 1881-1981: Collected Views of the Past: Haliburton, Ontario: Monmouth Historical Committee 1981.

Richard Pope. *Me N'Len*. Toronto and London: Dundurn Press, 1985

Nila Reynolds. *In Quest of Yesterday*. Minden, Ontario: The Provisional County of Haliburton, 1973.

Taylor Wilkins. *Haliburton By Rail and the I.B.&O.* Lindsay, Ontario: John Deyell Ltd. 1992.

Index

ABOUT THE AUTHOR

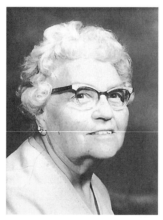

Gertrude Frances LeRoy Miller
(1902–1983)

Gertrude Frances LeRoy Miller was, in many ways, a woman ahead of her times. The skills, talents and leadership abilities she brought to the Wilberforce Outpost in September 1930 were well-honed before her arrival.

According to her sister, Virginia LeRoy Luckock, when the LeRoy family moved to Toronto in 1918, Gertrude "was a commercial artist for the United Drug Co., hand painting all the show cards (window ads) for Liggett and Rexall Drug Stores under the direction of Mr. George Howell. She took china-painting lessons and painted some beautiful pieces. Gert decided to become a missionary but when her plans didn't work out she decided on nursing."

She trained at Toronto Western Hospital, graduating with the Class of 1929 and received a scholarship to study Public Health Nursing at the University of Toronto.

Eager to begin applying her skills and knowledge, she accepted a call by the Canadian Red Cross (Ontario Division) to take charge of the one-nurse Outpost Hospital in Wilberforce, Ontario. This well-educated, well-trained, single, twenty-eight year old woman approached her nursing assignment with missionary zeal. Within days of her arrival, she had reorganized the office, storage area and patient rooms at the Outpost. She immediately began a program of regular visits to all the area schools, promoting hygiene to the children and checking their vision and hearing.

Accepted in the village for her nursing abilities, she must have been considered quite a groundbreaker. She bought her own car in 1931 and drove it everywhere. She used every means of transportation during winter when roads were covered with snow. She wore pants to keep warm on those cold winter treks to reach patients. She had all the up-to-date gadgets such as a flashlight and battery operated radio. She had Toronto newspapers mailed to her on the train three times a week.

Gertrude carried out her duties faithfully, but still had time for social activities which included dances at the Orange Hall, euchre parties, the annual Red Cross Picnic, Christmas Concerts and canoe rides with Del. Ultimately, she purchased a house which she called the "Cottage" so her family had a place of their own during their visits to be with her.

Her sister Virginia comments (October 1999): "I used to enjoy going up to the Outpost (from Toronto) to visit Gert. It was an all-day trip, even on the train, but we didn't mind. Gert was always glad to see us and Aileen (Ames) treated us royally. She was a wonderful cook as well as helping look after Gert, the patients and anything else that turned up. She is still a good friend and we correspond often. ... I know she [Gert] made the right decisions as she really loved being at the Outpost."

The Outpost, now a Historic House Museum, celebrates the lives of the many Red Cross Nurses who served there. None is celebrated more, in picture and artifacts, than Gertrude. Her contributions as nurse in the community are well remembered at the Outpost. This book, *Mustard Plasters and Handcars, Through the Eyes of a Red Cross Outpost Nurse* will be a lasting indication of Gertrude LeRoy Miller's life of devotion to her family, her community and her country.

Hilda Clark

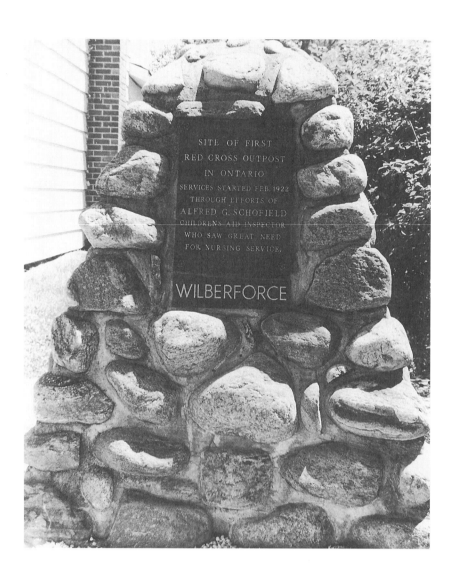

SITE OF FIRST
RED CROSS OUTPOST
IN ONTARIO
SERVICES STARTED FEB. 1922
THROUGH EFFORTS OF
ALFRED G. SCHOFIELD
CHILDRENS AID INSPECTOR
WHO SAW GREAT NEED
FOR NURSING SERVICE.

WILBERFORCE